Ignaz Semmelweis and the Vienna School of Medicine

By
Nicholas Kadar

Foreword by K. Codell Carter

Ignaz Semmelweis and the Vienna School of Medicine

By
Nicholas Kadar

Foreword by K. Codell Carter

Academica Press
Washington~London

Library of Congress Cataloging-in-Publication Data

Names: Kadar, Nicholas, author.
Title: Ignaz Semmelweis and the vienna school of medicine / Nicholas Kadar

Description: Washington : Academica Press, 2020. | Includes references.
Identifiers: LCCN 2020945285 | ISBN 9781680539486 (hardcover)

To the memory of my tutor, Dr. Victor Coxon

Contents

ABBREVIATIONS USED TO CITE TO PRIMARY AND SECONDARY SOURCES

Primary Sources

Brücke	Ernst Ritter von Brücke, *Sitzungsbericht der mathematisch-naturwisselschaftlichen Classe der Akademie der Wissenschaften zu Wien*, 1850, 7 (II), 291 (quoted in its entirety in Semmelweis's *Lehre* (vGy, 288-289)).
Ed.	Editorial, *Gazette Médicale de Paris* (1850) 3, (No. 5), pp. 382-383, available online: http://www.biusante.parisdescartes.fr/histmed/medica/page?90182x1850x05&p=382.
vGy	Tiberius von Györy, *Semmelweis' gesammelte Werke*, available on line at https://archive.org/stream/semmelweisgesam00semm goog#page/n7/mode/2up
K	Adolf Kussmaul, Adolf (1899). *Jugenderinnerungen eines alten Arztes*. (Berlin: Beliner Ausgabe, 2013).
M	Erna Lesky, *Ignaz Philipp Semmelweis und die Wiener Medizinische Schule* (Graz. Wien: H. Böhlau, 1964).
P	Erich Podach, "Die Entdeckung der Verursachung und Verhütbarkeit des Kindbettfiebers durch I. Ph. Semmelweis." *Ärztliche Wochenschrift* 1/2 (1947): 872-876.
SC	Ignaz Philipp Semmelweis, *The etiology, concept, and prophylaxis of childbed fever* (Madison: University of Wisconsin Press. Translated and edited by K. Codell Carter, 1983).
Skoda	Skoda, J (1849). Ueber die von Dr. Semmelweis entdeckte wahre Ursache der in der Wiener Gebäranstalt ungewöhlich häuftig vorkommenden Erkrankungen der Wöcherinnen und des Mittels zur Verminderung dieser Erkrankungen bis auf die gewöhliche Zahl. *Sitzungsberichte der mathematisch-*

	naturwissenschaftlichen Classe der Kaiserlichen Akademie der, 168-82. available online at: http:// www.zobodat.at/pdf/ SBAWW_03_0139-0186. pdf (also reproduced in von Gyory's compilation (vGy, 34-45)
SM	Ignaz Philipp Semmelweis, *The etiology, the concept, and the prophylaxis of childbed fever* (Birmingham: The Classics of Medicine Library, 351-478; 481-589; 591-715; 719-773. Translated by Frank P. Murphy, 1941).
Wieger	Friedrich Wieger, 'Des moyens prophylactiques mis en usage au grand hôpital de Vienne contre l'apparition de fièvre puerpérerale', *Gazette Médicale de Strasbourg* (1849)

Secondary Sources

B	István Benedek, *Ignaz Philipp Semmelweis (1818-1865)* (Wien-Köln-Grz: Hermann Böhlaus, 1983, Translated [from Hungarian to German] by Brigitte Engel).
C&C	K. Codell Carter & Barbara R. Carter, *Childbed fever: a scientific biography of Ignaz Semmelweis* (New Brunswick & London: Transaction Publishers, 2005).
G-Z	György Gortvay and Imre Zoltán, *Semmelweis: his life and work,* E Rona (Budapest: Akadémiai Kiadó, 1966. Translated by Éva Róna, revised translation by R. Bonnerjea, 1968).
Lesky	Erna Lesky, *The Vienna Medical School of the 19th Century* (Baltimore: Johns Hopkins University Press. Translated by L Williams and IS Levij, M.D, 1976).
R.	Mike Rappaport, 1848 Year of Revolution (New York: Basic Books, 2008)
vW	Fritz Schürer von Waldheim, Ignaz Philipp Semmelweis: Sein Leben und Wirken, (Wien und Leipzig: A. Hartleben's Verlag, 1905).
S.	William J. Sinclair, Semmelweis, *His Life and His Doctrine*, (Manchester: University of Machester Publications, 1909).

FOREWORD

Ignaz Semmelweis is famous for reducing the incidence of a particular disease, then called "childbed fever," that, in his day, ravaged the maternity wards of Vienna's General Hospital (the Allgemeines Krankenhaus—AKH). Semmelweis's work seems to receive more attention year by year, and everyone recognizes that it was among the pivotal accomplishments in the history of medicine. However, beyond that shared recognition, there is little agreement about many of the important issues having to do with Semmelweis's life and work.

Through the late twentieth century, Erna Lesky was among Austria's leading medical historians, and she devoted much of her professional career to recounting the history of the Vienna Medical School. In the course of her investigations, she discovered numerous documents, previously lost, concerning Semmelweis's relation to his professors and to the administrative officials who controlled his fate at the AKH. These documents are of keen interest, and Lesky performed a great service in bringing them to light. Based on the documents, Lesky wrote a monograph, *Ignaz Philipp Semmelweis und die Wiener Medizinische Schule*, in which she argued for various conclusions about Semmelweis's discoveries and about his relation to his colleagues at the AKH. Until now, Lesky's monograph, and, therefore, the original documents and her attempts to derive conclusions from them, has remained untranslated and relatively inaccessible. However, Lesky also wrote a monumental volume entitled *Die Wiener Medizinische Schule im 19. Jahrhundert*. This work has been translated and is readily available. Unfortunately, in this volume, the Semmelweis story is relegated to a very few pages; in those pages, Lesky repeats her conclusions from the Semmelweis monograph, but without the documents and without the arguments by which her views are supposedly justified. As a result, as things stand, her wide influence in matters pertaining to Semmelweis rests more on her personal reputation than on the documents and arguments that are, supposedly, the basis for her views.

Nicholas Kadar's translation of and commentary on Lesky's Semmelweis monograph is highly valuable in at least four ways: First, for the first time, it makes readily available, in English, many primary documents (not only those included in Lesky's monograph, but others as well) concerning Semmelweis's work and his relation to various officials and teachers at the AKH. Second, it provides an opportunity to appraise the arguments on which Lesky's widely accepted conclusions are based. Third, Kadar's commentary makes it quite obvious that Lesky's arguments are deeply flawed, and, therefore, that many of her influential opinions are, at the very least, inadequately supported, and, more likely, simply false. And, finally, Kadar's commentary also helps us follow, step by step, the process by which Semmelweis reached his conclusions; many details in this process has been in dispute but, as yet, no one has given as clear and as reasoned an account of those steps as has Kadar.

The documents that Lesky discovered provide clear and indisputable insight into some of the problems that Semmelweis encountered. Semmelweis conducted his work against a background of political disputes that began, in part, at the AKH and that culminated in the bloody riots of 1848. A central issue in those disputes was a power struggle between younger members of the medical faculty, men like Josef Skoda and Carl Rokitansky, and senior members such as Johann Klein, who was Semmelweis's chief in the first maternity clinic. Lesky's documents show clearly that Klein supported Semmelweis's work until Skoda sought to use Semmelweis's success to serve his (Skoda's) own interests and did so in such a way that, in Klein's opinion, undermined his (Klein's) own role as chief in the maternity clinic. At that point, unsurprisingly, Klein immediately withdrew his support, and Semmelweis's career at the AKH was doomed—doomed because of Skoda, whom Lesky identifies as "the main campaigner for Semmelweis." Was Skoda totally blind to the inevitable and disastrous consequences his behavior would have for Semmelweis, or was he simply indifferent to those consequences? At this point, there is no way to decided. But, either way, the very documents that Lesky provides, force one to seriously doubt the conclusions that she wants to draw from them.

This problem becomes especially acute when it comes to what Lesky refers to as "the methodical requirements of Semmelweis's discovery." In this section of her monograph, Lesky's main goal is to show that Skoda and Rokitansky should be recognized as sharing "spiritual co-authorship" [geistiger Miturheberschaft] in Semmelweis's discoveries; she wants, desperately, to shift credit for Semmelweis's discovery to his teachers in Vienna. Unfortunately, the evidence she provides points in precisely the opposite direction. Lesky claims that Semmelweis's work was based on a thorough mastery of contemporary pathological anatomy, on a particular kind of reasoning that has been referred to as "the elimination of factors," and on the use of statistical proof. No doubt, all of these were important to Semmelweis. But usually not in the way that Lesky seems to believe.

Semmelweis studied pathological anatomy with Rokitansky who was certainly among the world's leading contributors to that field. But Lesky herself points out that, for Semmelweis, his "years of training and experience in systematic pathological anatomical thinking" culminated in his (Semmelweis's) ability "to override the view of his teacher Rokitansky." Following the principles of pathological anatomy, Rokitansky divided childbed fever into a range of *different* diseases (depending on which tissues displayed morbidity)—Semmelweis emphatically rejected that view, that is, he rejected the implications of pathological anatomy, and instead, insisted that all cases of childbed fever were the same one disease. He did this, not on the basis of pathological anatomy, but on etiological grounds: they were all the same disease because they all shared a common cause. Such reasoning was absolutely inconsistent with the views held by both Skoda and Rokitansky. How, pray tell, can reaching a conclusion that *overrides*, that is, rejects, the views of one's teacher, secure that teacher in a role of "spiritual co-authorship" in one's conclusion? Surely, that makes no sense.

Lesky writes that "by combining [Skoda's] methods with Rokitansky's pathological-anatomical reasoning, and employing them ingeniously to solve his special question about the cause of the difference in mortality between the two divisions, [Semmelweis] attained a new synthesis: the discovery of the true cause of childbed fever." She then continues, "Skoda, with the inner evidence of spiritual co-authorship, immediately recognized in this [discovery a] new, genuine product of those methods of investigation and thought that Rokitansky and he had so distinctly imprinted on their school." But, if Skoda so clearly recognized Semmelweis's discovery as a "genuine product" of his own methods, and, indeed, as something in which he shared "spiritual co-authorship," how is one to explain the historical fact that never once, not even in lectures specifically on childbed fever, did Skoda ever accept Semmelweis's main conclusion that every case of the disease had one common cause? Again, Lesky would apparently have us believe that, reaching a conclusion exactly opposite to Skoda's somehow proves that Skoda was a "spiritual co-author" of Semmelweis's discovery. It seems much more likely that Lesky's desire to cast Semmelweis as entirely a product of the Vienna school blinded her to the recognition that Semmelweis's discovery was possible only after he completely *repudiated* many of the central principles that guided work at that school. All of this becomes absolutely clear in Kadar's marvelous commentary.

Through a meticulous analysis of the historical documents, including those unearthed by Lesky, Kadar also resolves numerous issues that have, so far, remained unclear. Here are two examples: first, what was the purpose of Semmelweis's animal experiments? Lesky takes for granted Skoda's suggestion that these experiments were conducted at his (Skoda's) suggestion in order to remove lingering doubts about Semmelweis's conclusions. Second, why did Semmelweis abruptly leave Vienna in October 1850? Lesky assumes that, thanks to Skoda's efforts, Semmelweis's request for a renewed appointment at the AKH was about to be granted, and, therefore, she finds his departure "incomprehensible." However, in both cases, Kadar provides strong evidence, based largely on a careful reading of the very documents that Lesky herself discovered, in support of Semmelweis's own explanations, and thereby shows that Lesky's conclusions are, at best, seriously misleading. Indeed, as Kadar observes, Lesky's account is "not an historical narrative at all" but an attempt to "use past events to illustrate . . . some matter of current concern," in this case, the current concern is proving that Semmelweis's brilliant innovation was the intellectual property of the Vienna School.

It remains only to observe that Kadar has lifted our understanding of Semmelweis to an entirely new level. From this point on, no one engaged in Semmelweis research can be excused for failing to study Kadar's translation and commentary of Lesky's monograph, not only to clarify many aspects of Semmelweis's life and work, but still more as a safeguard against falling into popular yet unwarranted misconceptions that are still widely promulgated.

K. Codell Carter
Provo, Utah.

INTRODUCTION

Anyone who speaks only English and tries to understand how the Hungarian obstetrician, Ignaz Philipp Semmelweis (1818-1865) discovered the cause and prophylaxis of childbed fever, is faced with the insurmountable problem that most primary documents probative of this question are written in German, Hungarian, French and Danish, and only a few have been translated into English.[1] Consequently, although the Anglo-American literature on Semmelweis is extensive, almost all of it is based on secondary sources that accept, without critically examining, secondary-source answers to very important questions about Semmelweis and his work,[2] not the least of which is how Semmelweis was led to his discovery, and why his theory received such a hostile reception in Vienna, where Semmelweis was the Assistant on the first maternity division of the Vienna General Hospital (*Allgemeines Krankenhaus*-AKH).

The pre-eminent historian of the Vienna Medical School of that era was the Austrian historian Erna Lesky (1911-1986), who was honored for her extraordinary productivity with a *Festschrifft* on her seventieth birthday,[3] and whose magnum opus, *The Vienna Medical School of the Nineteenth Century* was published on the centennial of Semmelweis's death in 1965, and translated into English in 1976. However, Lesky's historiography of Semmelweis was published a year earlier, in a separate monograph, *Ignaz Philipp Semmelweis und die Wiener Medizinische Schule*, that has never been translated into English, notwithstanding that Nikolaus Mani concluded his review of Lesky's monograph with "whoever deals with Semmelweis must read E. Lesky's book. The reviewer thinks that this fundamental study should also be available in English."[4]

[1] Kadar & Croft, 2020, p.1.

[2] Loudon; Nuland (1979, 1995, 2003); Obenchain.

[3] Ganzinger, et al .

[4] Mani, p. 390.

Lesky's monograph had its origins in a decision by the Austrian Academy of Sciences to establish a 'Commission for the History of the Natural Sciences,' of which Lesky was one of the Commissioners. The Commission compiled a series of publications captioned, "Publications of the Commission for the History of Mathematics and the Natural Sciences," and Lesky's monograph was the first publication in the series. In that monograph Lesky published important documents for the first time that Lesky herself had discovered in the Austrian archives ("Lesky Documents"). The Lesky Documents had been overlooked by the Austrian historian Fritz Schürer von Waldheim in his biography of Semmelweis,[5] and their discovery corrected important errors in Waldheim's biography on which English biographers later relied.[6] The documents Lesky discovered were translated into Hungarian and donated by the Vienna Medical School to the Semmelweis University in Budapest in 1973,[7] but, like Lesky's monograph itself, they have never been translated into English.

The documents Lesky discovery have shed important new light on what happened to Semmelweis in Vienna, and specifically on: (1) the relationship between Semmelweis and his chief, Johann Klein; (2) the opposition Semmelweis's theory faced from Klein and others at the AKH where Semmelweis worked as the Assistant on the first maternity division (*Klinik*) for twenty-eight tumultuous months (from July 1, 1846 to March 20, 1849, with a five-month break from October 20, 1846); (3) why Semmelweis abruptly left Vienna in mid-October, 1850; and (4) why Semmelweis likely felt he was in no position to publish his work until he had collected further clinical evidence in support of his theory, long after he left Vienna. The unavailability of these documents in English has, therefore, redounded significantly to the detriment of the Anglo-American literature on Semmelweis.

Unfortunately, however, Lesky's monograph did not address these questions, much less elucidate the presuppositions, empirical observations, and the rationale of the inferences that led Semmelweis to

---

[5] von Waldheim.
[6] Sinclair; Slaughter.
[7] Lesky (1973).

his discovery and caused him to conduct animal experiments with Rokitansky's Assistant, Georg Maria Lautner, in 1849. Instead, Lesky's narrative obfuscated these questions by claiming that Semmelweis's discovery entailed nothing more than the application of the methodology Semmelweis had learned from Joseph Skoda (1805-1881) in a new context, and by rejecting Semmelweis's own account of his discovery and substituting for it an account that arrogated to Skoda and the Vienna Medical School much of the credit for the discovery that belonged to Semmelweis alone.

Although Lesky's monograph has never been translated into English, her reconstruction of Semmelweis's discovery made its way into the English historiography via her *magnum opus*, in which Lesky wrote:

> It has been overlooked that in arriving at his causality, Semmelweis used a particular method of reasoning which was peculiar to the later Vienna Medical School. We need only recall Skoda's method of exclusion…in order to realize that it was this very method that Semmelweis adopted, the method of exclusion with its strict, step-by-step procedure of modus tollendo ponens. Semmelweis had learned how to apply its technique when he attended Skoda's lectures and he used it successfully in solving the problem that had aroused his special interest, i.e. in finding the cause of the higher mortality at the physicians' clinic.
>
> It was not by mere chance, therefore, that Semmelweis's theory formed the subject of Skoda's lecture to the Academy of Sciences in 1849. Step by step Skoda retraced the way in which Semmelweis had arrived at his discovery, and at the same time used this brilliant application on the part of his disciple as a classic example for demonstrating his own method of thinking, the method per exclusionem. (Lesky, 185-186)

Given Lesky's stature as a historian, these assertions were accepted uncritically as accurate, and Lesky's narrative of Skoda's relationship to Semmelweis's discovery has become an integral part of the English historiography of Semmelweis even though Lesky's account finds little support in historical facts.

For one thing, as the philosopher, Codell Carter has pointed out, far from retracing "step by step…the way in which Semmelweis had arrived at his discovery" as Lesky claimed, Skoda never accepted Semmelweis's theory of childbed fever, and his account was in at least two respects, "incompatible with the account that Semmelweis ultimately gave,"[8] and "attributed to Semmelweis a view that he [Skoda] himself found more acceptable than Semmelweis's own true position."[9]

For another thing, after excluding all the putative causes of childbed fever—epidemic causes, the seasons, overcrowding, fear, the position in which women delivered—Semmelweis was able to deduce only what did *not* cause childbed fever, and nothing at all about its actual cause, and which left Semmelweis dejectedly lamenting, "Everything was uncertain, everything was doubtful, everything was inexplicable, only the enormous number of deaths was an indubitable fact." (SM, 390).

The Hungarian scholar, Jozsef Antall, also subsequently showed that it is far from clear that Semmelweis even learned about the disjunctive syllogism from Skoda because Jozsef Purgstaller, a member of the Hungarian Academy of Sciences, who held a doctorate in philosophy and had published a book "Rudiments of Philosophy," taught at the high school (gymnasium) Semmelweis had attended in Buda, and specifically this syllogism, and after high school Semmelweis also took 'two classes in philosophy' at the University of Pest, where Purgstaller also taught, before he enrolled in the Vienna Medical School.[10] Moreover, the concluding sentence of Semmelweis's book, *The Aetiology, Concept and Prophylaxis of Childbed Fever* (*Aetiology*), suggests that he had taken "courses on logic" for he admonished Carl Braun, who succeeded Semmelweis as Assistant, and then Klein as Professor on the first maternity division, "not to neglect to take some semesters of logic as soon as possible." (SM 771)

Never the less, Lesky's narrative continues to be repeated by English-speaking biographers who have based their accounts on Lesky's

---

[8] Carter (1984), p. 341.
[9] Ibid., pp. 340-342.
[10] Antall, pp. 119-120.

representations about Semmelweis's discovery in her *magnum opus*. For example, in a recent (2016) biography Obenchain wrote:

> Skoda envisioned something more than just a revolutionary theory. Semmelweis's great generalization, his entire inductive scheme, was a prime example of New School methodology... Skoda sensed not only a grand opportunity to advance theoretical scientific medicine, but also to improve the image of the New School at the same time...In January, 1849, Skoda delivered a major address to Vienna's Committee of Professors in which he celebrated his young mentee as a prime example of someone who had learned and employed the modern scientific method to solve a major enigma...Skoda led his assemblage step by step along Semmelweis's path to enlightenment, accenting his use of statistics and *per exclusionem* as his primary methods of logic.[11]

And, although Obenchain accepted Carter's proof that "[t]here is no evidence that Skoda ever split from orthodoxy, remaining a committed multicausalist throughout his career,"[12] he never questioned Lesky's narrative:

> Whatever his reasons may have been, Skoda treaded that narrow line, speaking in favour of the *Lehre* while continuing to believe in the multicausalism. For Skoda and his war on the medieval Old School, Semmelweis's triumphant elucidation of the puerperal fever question represented too great an opportunity to squander over some theoretical disagreement.[13]

Therefore, I undertook this translation and critique of Lesky's monograph to make accessible to readers and students of Semmelweis who speak only English the primary documents without which an accurate understanding of Semmelweis's actions, and of what happened to him in Vienna, cannot be gained. I have appended translations of the texts of three additional documents not included in Lesky's monograph as these are also critical to the understanding what happened to Semmelweis in Vienna:

---

[11] Obenchain, p. 103.
[12] Obenchain, p. 104.
[13] Ibid., 105.

Skoda's October 18, 1849 lecture to the Academy of Sciences on Semmelweis's work (Appendix A); Brücke's memorandum to the Academy dated October 31, 1850 (Appendix B); and the Minutes of the May 15, 1850 Metting of the Society of Physicians at which Semmelweis delivered a lecture describing his research (Appendix C). In my overview and critique of Lesky's account, I present and discuss events that Lesky did not discuss or omitted entirely, and that are crucial to understanding what happened to Semmelweis in Vienna, such as the animal experiments Semmelweis conducted with Rokitansky's assistant, Georg Maria Lautner in 1849, and with the preeminent physiologist of his day, Erns Ritter von Brüke, in 1850. My purpose in doing so is to provide information about all the events related to Semmelweis's professional activities while he was in Vienna and thereby allow readers to draw their own informed conclusions about what really happened to Semmelweis in Vienna before he returned to Pest in October, 1850.

I have paraphrased some of parts of Lesky monograph because of uncertainties over copyright ownership, but since copyright law only protects modes of expression, and not the ideas or facts expressed, the paraphrased translations contain all the ideas and facts contained in the original. The archival documents (and the material in the appendices) have been translated in their entirety, as have Lesky's most important claims, as she wrote them, to assure the reader that the claims imputed to Lesky are ones she actually made and not my interpretations of what she wrote. Non-paraphrased translations have been placed in single quotation marks; translations of material quoted by Lesky are placed in double quotation marks.

ACKNOWLEDGEMENT

This work stands squarely on the shoulders of the enormous original contributions that the philosopher Codell Carter has made to the historiography of Semmelweis. Carter is not only the most insightful living Semmelweis scholar, he is the only contemporary English-speaking biographer of Semmelweis who has based his work entirely on primary sources. Carter broke entirely new ground by elucidating the causal reasoning underlying Semmelweis's discovery, and by showing that it likely influenced the rise of germ theory of disease, and development of modern concept of medicine.

This work would also not have been possible but for the invitation from Dr. Roberto Romero, Editor-in-Chief for Obstetrics of the *American Journal of Obstetrics and Gynecology*, to commemorate the bicentennial of Semmelweis's birth with an article summarizing Semmelweis's life and work.[14] That undertaking made me realize how little of the contemporary Anglo-American Semmelweis literature was based on primary sources, but time constraints precluded me from retrieving, much less translating all the primary sources from which I have constructed the history summarized in the present critique of Lesky's historiography of Semmelweis.

I am also indebted to Dr. Russell Dominic Croft for translating two critical documents for me from the French that, in conjunction with Carter's translation of Hermann Schwartz's letter to Michaelis, and the text of some of the documents Lesky discovered in the Austrian archives, elucidated for the first time the logical objections that Semmelweis's theory and proof faced from his chief and others at the AKH, and that had prompted Semmelweis to conduct animal experiments with Lautner in 1849. These two articles were (1) Frederick Wieger's article published on

[14] Kadar (2019).

April 20, 1849 in the *Gazette Médicale de Strasbourg*, which reported for the first time the annual maternal mortality rates from childbed fever on the first maternity division of the AKH for the years 1841-1848, and the results of Semmelweis's chlorine hand-disinfection experiment, and (2) an Editorial in the *Gazette Médicale de Paris* commenting on, and questioning the significance of the results of the chlorine hand-disinfection experiment that Wieger had reported.[15]

Finally, I have dedicated this work to my tutor, the late Dr. Victor Coxon, Reader in Physiology at Oxford University, because his lasting influence on me is ultimately responsible for this work. Dr. Coxon always insisted that I read the original sources of the principles he wanted me to learn, even when they were experiments from the nineteenth century, and it was the habit of mind he thus inculcated in me that left me so dissatisfied with the information I was able to glean from secondary sources about Semmelweis's work. Dr. Coxon also always admonished me to be my own worst devil's advocate, and I hope I have succeeded in holding fast to this principle as well in my overview and critique of Professor Lesky's narrative of Semmelweis's Vienna years.

---

[15] Kadar & Croft.

OVERVIEW

Semmelweis's discovery of the cause and prophylaxis of childbed fever was deemed by the historian Fielding Garrison to be "the greatest single achievement of a member of the New Vienna Medical School," (FG, 435), and Lesky considered it "one of the greatest discoveries in the history of medicine" [**M, 7**]. Yet, Lesky's monograph is not really about the history of Semmelweis's discovery at all. It does not cite or quote a single sentence from Semmelweis's *Aetiology*; it does not mention the empirical observations on which Semmelweis based his inferences, much less the logic or presuppositions of those inferences; and it does not describe or summarize Semmelweis's own account of his discovery. On the contrary, Lesky dismissed Semmelweis's own account of his discovery as an after-the-fact reconstruction based on earlier work by the Hungarian-born, Nietzsche scholar, Eric Podach (1894-1967), [**M, 56-57**] even though the factual premise of Podach's argument—that Semmelweis did not have sufficient autopsy experience to have made the anatomico-pathological connections when he said he made them—was not correct, (Lesky,141, 185), and the first-hand, eyewitness account in Adolf Kussmaul's memoirs confirmed Semmelweis's own account of how he was led to his discovery. (K, 173-174).

Nominally, Lesky's monograph is about the documents she discovered in the Austrian archives that shed new light on events that affected Semmelweis's career in Vienna. These were:

(1) Semmelweis's application for a two-year extension of his assistantship on December 1, 1848, and appeal from the denial of that application (of which Semmelweis was only notified on March 19, 1849, the last day of his assistantship);

(2) Skoda's motion to the medical College of Professors on January 16, 1849, asking the College to appoint a commission to investigate why the maternal mortality rate (MMR) from

childbed fever on the first maternity division of the AKH had dropped so dramatically after chlorine hand-disinfection was implemented at the end of May, 1847 ("Skoda's motion");

(3) Semmelweis's application for *habilitation* and docentur on February 9, 1850, and re-application for a docentur on May 9, 1850 following the denial of his first application on April 2, 1850;

(4) Semmelweis's nomination to replace his chief, Johann Klein, as Professor of Obstetrics of the first maternity division, following Klein's death in April, 1856.

The historical narrative Lesky constructed based on these documents was also not primarily concerned with what happened to Semmelweis in Vienna but, rather, to chronicle the depth of support Semmelweis enjoyed from progressive members of the Vienna Medical School throughout his time in Vienna, and even after he left Vienna, when they proposed that Semmelweis be appointed to succeed Klein's as professor on the first maternity division of the AKH. Lesky did not probe the consequences of this involvement by members of the Vienna Medical School in Semmelweis's research, and instead asked a question the documents she discovered could not answer: what role did the Vienna Medical School play in Semmelweis's discovery? Her answer, which did not come from those documents, was that most of the credit for Semmelweis's discovery actually belonged to Skoda and the New Vienna Medical School:

> However, we want to bring Semmelweis back into the milieu of his school and the ground from which his discovery grew, and confront the often-discussed question of what Vienna owes Semmelweis and compare it with what he owed to Vienna's medical school. The answer can only be: from a scientific point of view, all the methodological means that were a prerequisite for his discovery. [**M-56**].

But Lesky did not stop at claiming that Semmelweis learned all 'the methodological prerequisites' necessary for his discovery from Skoda and the Vienna Medical School: she declared Semmelweis's discovery to be the intellectual property of the Vienna Medical School, and Skoda, effectively, to be its co-author:

> Skoda, with the inner evidence of **spiritual co-authorship** [*geistiger Miturheberschaft*], immediately recognized in this new, genuine product of those methods of investigation and thought that Rokitansky and he had so distinctly imprinted on their school…[and] felt, to the highest degree, responsible to science and humanity, to ensure that **this intellectual property of the Viennese school** took its place in science and obstetrical practice. [**M, 61**, boldface added].

Lesky even credited the Vienna Medical School for the acclaim Semmelweis received for his lecture to the Society of Physicians on his discovery on May 15, 1850, and declared it "the first major success of the Vienna School in its fight for Semmelweis." [**M, 77]**

Lesky portrayed Semmelweis's supporters at the Vienna Medical School as constantly fighting, battling, campaigning or struggling for Semmelweis and his discovery, and Skoda, "the main campaigner for Semmelweis," [**M, 55**], as "Semmelweis's teacher" or "master," and even as "Semmelweis's lawyer" (*Amwalt*) [**M, 19**], and referred to Semmelweis always as Skoda's "student" or "pupil." She construed each event involving Semmelweis as part of the Vienna Medical School's overarching struggle on behalf of Semmelweis's discovery, and placed responsibility for Semmelweis's professional fate in Vienna solely on Semmelweis, "the incomprehensible waverer" [**M, 64**], the only one [who] did not show up in the bitter struggle for **the greatest discovery of the Vienna School**…[**M, 51**, boldface added], and who, incomprehensibly, "escaped from Vienna" in mid-October, 1850. But the historical facts Lesky omitted from her narrative, coupled with those in the very documents she discovered, paint an entirely different picture: that Skoda cost Semmelweis his job, and caused Semmelweis and his theory more harm than any of his opponents ever did.

The undoing of Semmelweis's career in Vienna began with Skoda's motion to the medical College of Professors on January 16, 1849. This was revealed by the information contained in the Lesky Documents for they clearly indicate that Skoda's motion turned Klein against

Semmelweis, and caused Klein to change his mind about extending Semmelweis's assistantship for another two years. Lesky admitted as much:

> Between November 19, 1848 and January 20, 1849, Klein made a disastrous about turn and changed his mind about extending Semmelweis's assistantship ...[and] first became Semmelweis's opponent in this fight. [**M-49**]

But Lesky tried to divest Skoda's motion of its consequences. She argued that although Semmelweis's application and Skoda's motion involved separate administrative procedures, it was inevitable that Skoda's motion would have 'a retroactive effect on Semmelweis's application,' but the faculty's moral obligation to promote and disseminate medical knowledge obligated it to conduct the 'scientific examination of Semmelweis's discovery' that Skoda was proposing. **[M-19]** Indeed, she claimed that 'the whole extent of the struggle for Semmelweis' could only be understood if one grasped the inextricable connection that existed between Skoda's motion and Semmelweis's application, as if this was all somehow unavoidable, and that it would be unfair not to see this necessary connection or interpret Skoda's motion in any other way—in other words, unfair to blame Skoda for what happened to Semmelweis:

> Only such a synoptic view allows one to see that both the arguments about Skoda's motion and the extension of Semmelweis's assistantship were used in the great struggle of a school out of whose soil Semmelweis's discovery grew. Equity requires that this struggle of the Viennese Medical School be given its rightful place in the history of medicine. [**M, 36**].

But there was no necessary connection whatsoever between the two events. Lesky conceded that if Skoda had not intervened, Klein would have granted Semmelweis's request for an extension of his assistantship, and that one could deduce from Klein and Bartsch's later reports that Semmelweis sought to extend his assistantship as 'only extension of his service gave him the opportunity to prove without any doubt the success of the previous chlorine washings.' **[M-19]**. And what Lesky never explained is why, even assuming the medical faculty had the moral obligation to promote and disseminate medical knowledge Skoda imputed to it, this necessitated Skoda to request that a commission be appointed to investigate exactly the same question as Semmelweis sought an extension of his assistantship to investigate.

Skoda's motion and Semmelweis's request for an extension were only connected temporally, and only because both were, in different and unconnected ways, consequences of the riots that were triggered by the Emperor's sending of troops to quell the uprising in Hungary on October 6, 1848. The October riots were suppressed after five days of bloody fighting that began on October 26, 1848, during which Field Marshal Windisch-Grätz laid siege to Vienna. (R, 280, 285-287), and all the circumstantial evidence to be discussed in more detail later suggests that Semmelweis had planned to conduct animal experiments with Lautner at about this time in order to prove that not only could he prevent childbed fever by eliminating its putative cause, but he could also induce it, or at least pathological changes indistinguishable from it, in newly-delivered rabbits by introducing material from cadavers into their genital tracts. However, Lautner took part in the October riots and was arrested. [**M, 80**], and, therefore, Semmelweis's applied instead for an extension of his assistantship on December 1, 1848, in order that he might continue his research on childbed fever.[16] [**M, 43**]

Six weeks later, the same riots prompted Skoda to make his motion to the College of Professors in order to test whether the independence the College had been granted from the Ministry of Education earlier in the year still had force. Under the rules and regulations governing education within the Habsburg monarchy laid down by Stifft in 1804, the university faculty had no independence from the Ministry of Education over educational matters. (Lesky, 19) The liberal-minded Baron von Türkheim, who replaced Stifft in 1836, loosened these regulations, as did his successor Feuchtesleben in 1846, after Türkheim's death, [**M-13**] but even under the more relaxed rules, the faculty had no autonomy from the Ministry, which still decided all faculty appointments, prescribed how students were to be examined, and what curriculum they were to be taught. (Lesky, 96-104) All that changed on March 12, 1848, when riots erupted in Vienna, and students and young, liberal-minded faculty demanded

[16] Kadar (2020).

changes in the regulations under the slogan 'Freedom of Teaching and Freedom of Learning.' The Ministry granted these demands on March 30, 1848, and new regulations were drafted and submitted to the Ministry on April 12, 1848, but they were never ratified or put into effect. (Lesky, 96) The bloody suppression of the October riots called into question the gains made by the faculty towards self-governance and independence, and Skoda's proposal was calculated to test whether the independence granted to the College of Professors following the March riots still had force: Semmelweis and his research were merely the instrumentalities with which to achieve this objective.

That Skoda's motion turned Klein against Semmelweis, and was the direct cause of him denying Semmelweis's application for an extension of his assistantship was placed beyond doubt by the very documents Lesky herself had discovered in the Austrian archives. Indeed, as already noted, Lesky acknowledged that "Klein first became Semmelweis's opponent in this fight," i.e. the fight over Skoda's motion [**M-49**], and she concluded that before Skoda made his proposal Klein must have agreed to extend Semmelweis's appointment, as he had, by Klein's own admission, given Semmelweis a favourable reference on November 19, 1848—less than three weeks after Windisch-Grätz had quelled the October riots. There was also no one in training ready to take over from Semmelweis when his appointment came to an end on March 19, 1849, [**M-49**] nor were there any qualified applicants, and it was customary to require successful candidates to have up to six months training in obstetrics before they assumed their positions as assistant. [**M-41, 42**] Klein may not have accepted Semmelweis's conclusions about the effectiveness of chlorine hand-disinfection, but he had, after all, authorized its implementation, and had to have been pleased that the mortality rate on his division had fallen, whatever the reason. Moreover, Klein did not initially oppose Skoda's proposal. He only opposed it after he was excluded from the commission selected to investigate his own department; and Lesky acknowledged that it would have been reasonable for Klein to have assumed that he would be appointed chairman of the committee, or at least be one of its members, [**M, 23**], and that if the faculty was given authority "to intervene in the sphere of each individual member" it would create serious conflicts. [**M, 28**] In other words, Skoda had put Klein in an untenable position.

Skoda next involved himself in Semmelweis's research by delivering a lecture on Semmelweis's discovery before the Academy of Sciences on October, 18, 1849, and its consequences for Semmelweis were equally disastrous. It had been recognized long before Lesky wrote her monograph that Skoda created serious misunderstandings about Semmelweis's theory with this lecture by referring only to cadavers as the source of the agent causing childbed-fever. In 1905, Schürer von Waldheim wrote in his biography of Semmelweis:

> Skoda… spoke in general about "rotting animal substances"… but added that Semmelweis had recognized "the only possible way of transferring a rotting animal substance to the birth canals (*Geburtstelle*) of labouring women (*Wöchnerinnen*)" was by doctors who had been involved in autopsies. This was incorrect, this was Semmelweis's original point of view, which he soon recognized to be only one of the ways. But the fallacy of cadaver-infection as the only possible cause had been made and it spread out (*flatterte*) into the world. (vW, 53-54).

Lesky avoided confronting the damage that Skoda's lecture caused Semmelweis and his theory by simply ignoring entirely what Skoda had actually told the Academy of Sciences about Semmelweis's discovery: she did not quote a single sentence from the text of the lecture besides its title. Carter's scholarship took a giant step in advancing our understanding of Skoda's relationship to Semmelweis's discovery by pointing out for the first time that Skoda did not actually agree with Semmelweis's theory of the cause of childbed fever, and gave an entirely different account of the inferences that led to Semmelweis's discovery from the one Semmelweis himself later gave,[17] but because Carter's primary interest was in the genesis of modern concepts of disease, and the role that Semmelweis's conception of causation may have had in its genesis,[18] he did not explore the ramifications of Skoda's statements to the Academy for Semmelweis further.

---

[17] Carter (1984), p. 341.
[18] Carter (1985 & 2003).

Instead of analysing the text of Skoda's lecture, Lesky simply asserted that Semmelweis had learned the methodology she claimed he used to make his discovery from Skoda, and supported her contention not with historical evidence, but by asserting that a very special, student-teacher relationship existed between Semmelweis and Skoda (that actually existed between Semmelweis and Rokitansky, as described later), and which Lesky claimed explained why Skoda had 'adopted Semmelweis's discovery as if it was his own business.' **[M-55]** According to Lesky, 'Semmelweis was Skoda's pupil in the very pristine sense of the word.' As a student, Semmelweis had been 'one of the most eager visitors to Skoda's lectures,' had attended Skoda's medical department and associated division of chest diseases for almost a year and a half, and after Skoda was appointed professor in 1846, most wanted to be Skoda's assistant. This is how Semmelweis learned the method of exclusion that Lesky claimed was the cornerstone of the methodology Semmelweis used to make his discovery. **[M-58]**

Lesky characterized Skoda's lecture to the Academy as the beginning of "a new large-scale offensive for Semmelweis" [**M, 55**], whose

> tactical purpose…in the battle for Semmelweis [had] the same purpose as Haller's lecture to the Society of Physicians on February 23rd: to demonstrate in front of the world the importance of Semmelweis's discovery, and to give special emphasis to where it took place by the demonstration. [But] it was more than just a presentation, also more than a prelude to a new offensive: as Skoda traced, step by step, the path to Semmelweis's discovery (*Erkenntnisweg*) in front of the Academy, **he demonstrated at the same time a classic example of the ingenious application of his own method of working and thinking.** [**M, 62**, boldface added]

Indeed. The title of Skoda's lecture may have been, *"Regarding Dr. Semmelweis's Discovery of the True Cause of the Unusually High Incidence of Sickness among the Patients of the Viennese Maternity Hospital and the Means of Reducing This Incidence to Normal Levels,"* (vGy, 36), but the lecture was not so much about Semmelweis, much less the beginning of a new offensive fought on his behalf by his friends, as about Skoda himself: the doubts he had about Semmelweis's theory, the proposal he had ostensibly made to the medical College of Professors for resolving those doubts, and the doubts that he believed still remained—after more than eighteen months—about Semmelweis's theory.

It is difficult if not impossible to reconcile the second and last paragraphs of the text of Skoda's lecture with the view that he had intended with his lecture to begin a new offensive on behalf of Semmelweis, or delivered it for the tactical purpose of 'demonstrating to the world the importance of Semmelweis's discovery,' for the second paragraph of the text states:

> For the moment I will discuss the facts and conclusions from whose combination the discovery has arisen, and then *report on the measures, which seemed necessary to put the discovery beyond doubt*. (vGy, 36; Appendix A, p. 161, italics added).

In other words, at the very outset of his lecture, Skoda told the Academy that doubts remained about Semmelweis's theory, and that he was going describe what was still required to place the theory beyond all doubt. That Skoda was referring to himself when describing what "seemed necessary to put the discovery beyond doubt" is clear from the fact that each measure which this proof purportedly required was, Skoda claimed, recommended to Semmelweis by Skoda himself. (vGy, 41-42) Skoda enumerated these purported requirements under subheading B of his lecture, which was captioned:

> I find the measures that seemed necessary, *and that still seem necessary* to put Dr. Semmelweis's discovery beyond all doubt, to be the following. (vGy, 40; Appendix A, p. 167, italics added)

Skoda made four recommendations, the most important of which, he said, was the fourth, the recommendation to conduct animal experiments. (vGy, 41-2; SM, 607) It is, therefore, worth noting that Lesky did not say a word about Semmelweis's animal experiments, and never connected them with or construed them as a response to the objections that were raised about Semmelweis's theory by Klein or others at the AKH. Her only comment on the animal experiments was to point out that they could not have occupied all of Semmelweis's time between the end of his assistantship on March 19, 1849 and his returned to Pest in October, 1850: 'It is impossible for the nine animal experiments that Skoda referred to in his lecture to the Academy to have filled his time.' [**M, 52**]

Skoda claimed that he had made the four recommendations to the medical College of Professors in January, and although they were adopted by a majority of the College, the Ministry of Education intervened at Klein's request, and the investigation was never conducted. Therefore, Skoda claimed that he had asked Semmelweis to conduct the animal experiment that Semmelweis had already conducted with Lautner ("Lautner experiments") by the time Skoda delivered his lecture to the Academy of Sciences on October 18, 1849:

> The proposal was accepted by a majority of the College of Professors, and a Commission was immediately named; only the Ministry ruled on an objection from the Professor of obstetrics, that a commission hearing should not take place. As a result of this decision, I asked Dr. Semmelweis that he himself undertake experiments in animals. If these are attained the other tasks are of less importance. (vGy, 42; Appendix A, p. 168)

However, the minutes of the January 16, 1849 meeting give no indication that Skoda's proposal for the appointment of a commission included a recommendation that the commission investigate the four questions he outlined in his lecture to the Academy. On the contrary, the minutes state specifically that Skoda proposed that 'three-to-five members of the College be selected without delay **to investigate the relationship between the two maternity clinics**' and nothing at all about animal experiments. [**M-21**] Entirely consistent with this is the following statement in Skoda's response to Klein's objection to his proposal in which Skoda reaffirmed that the commission was asked to investigate specifically the cause of the difference in MMR between the two maternity divisions and not all the causes of childbed fever:

> The fact that the disease also occurred on the second maternity clinic could not be used as an objection to this supposition, as for the time being this was not treated as an issue about clarifying all the causes of childbed fever, but merely about

> finding out and preventing the root cause of the disproportionately high mortality on the first maternity clinic. **[M, 27]**

Skoda never explained either to the College of Professors or the Academy of Sciences what doubts about Semmelweis's theory the animal experiments he had ostensibly recommended were intended to resolve or how they could resolve them. And casting further doubt on Skoda's claim that the Lautner experiments were conducted at his suggestion is that these experiments had already been conducted by the time Skoda delivered his lecture to the Academy of Sciences, yet he was now telling the Academy of Sciences that the unspecified doubts they were intended to resolve remained, and that still "further, and more varied experiments" were required to resolve those remaining doubts—only, again, Skoda did not specify what those still remaining doubts were or how a fresh set of animal experiments could resolve them.

Skoda did point out that the Lautner experiments had a theoretical flaw—a greater quantity of putrid matter was introduced into the birth canals of the animals than could be left on the hands of the attendants after they had washed their hands with soap and water, which was the practice before chlorine hand-disinfection was implemented:

> One could object that in the experiments just cited a greater quantity of putrefying matter was involved, and that in eight cases the putrid substance was brought into contact with the birth-parts of the animals for several days, one after another, and once in only one case, whereas the quantity clinging to the hands—whatever it may be—must be considered very small, as the hands are always washed with water after examination of cadavers. (vGy, 45; Appendix A, p. 172)

However, Skoda himself dismissed this potential objection by saying that it 'seems to me to have no special weight,' (vGy, 45, Appendix A, p172), but nevertheless asked the Academy to award Semmelweis a grant to conduct additional experiments to dispel any remaining doubts about his theory—only this time to conduct the experiments with a member of the Academy to ensure that they were done properly (sic):

> Therefore, I ask that you be willing to support Dr. Semmelweis in further experiments with a grant of money, and in view of this, in order to dispel any doubts as to the correctness of the experiments, that these attempts be also made by a member of the Academy, and I ask Professor Brücke to undertake this task. (vGy, 45, Appendix A, p. 173)

Given the tenuous nature of Skoda's justification for conducting additional animal experiments, and his insistance that doubts remained about Semmelweis's theory, it is difficult to interpret Skoda determination to force Semmelweis to conduct further animal experiments as anything but an attempt to make it appear that Skoda had something to do with Semmelweis's discovery, and therefore to take part credit for it. This conclusion is rendered all the more compelling by the fact that a month or two after Skoda's lecture to the Academy of Sciences, Carl Haller, in his annual report on the AKH,[19] presented the results of the cholorine hand-disinfection experiment and said that the Lautner experiments had established Semmelweis's conclusion from the chlorine hand-disinfection experiment 'beyond all doubt:'

> And what is imperatively impressed upon the unprejudiced examiner of these figures [i.e. the annual MMR on the First and Second Divisions of the AKH for the years 1839-1848], has been established beyond all doubt by direct experiments on animals (injections of pus and ichor into the vaginae of newly delivered rabbits), which were done by Drs. Semmelweis and

[19] Haller's report was likely published in November or December, 1848. The date is not on the report, and Dr. Hermann Zeitlhofer, Librarian at the Viennese Society of Physicians graciously provided me with the following explanation:
"Nowhere in this volume the exact month in which the Haller-"Bericht" was published is stated. To prove that, I also attach the scan of the 'Content' of the volume ("Sachtregister") and a scan of the 'Left page of the first page of Hallers Bericht". On the left page you can see the date '9 November 1849'– so maybe 'Hallers Bericht' was published in November or December 1849. In the last line of the first page of Hallers Bericht you also can read "Z. d. W. Ä. 1848/49 VIII" – which maybe means: 'Zeitschrift der Wiener Ärzte 1848/49, VIII issue.' Also the high page number (starting with p. 493) would indicate that it was not early in the year 1849."

> Lautner recently, and should be publishede after full conclusion. (vGy, 35)[20]

Benedek summed it all up by pointing out that even if Skoda had done all this with good intentions it was nevertheless the case that:

> If the replies (*Antwortbriefe*) of Michaelis, Tilanus, Routh and others weren't available, we could not really decide what Semmelweis and what Skoda had discovered. The "liberality" (*Grossmütigkeit*) with which Skoda portrayed the insight into blood poisoning [i.e. that childbed fever was a form of blood poisoning and not a specific diseases of the puerperium as Rokitansky thought] as a joint discovery, made it possible for the Viennese medical historians...to transfer the credit [for Semmelweis's discovery] more and more onto the Skoda-Rokitanskhy-School. (B, 138).

Semmelweis conducted additional animal experiments with Brücke ("Brücke experiments") at the behest of Skoda in the spring and summer of 1850. The details of the experiments are not known. However, it is known from Brücke's memorandum to the Academy, dated October 31, 1850, that the experiments yielded only ambiguous results, and, more importantly, that Brücke, the leading physiologist of his day, had himself concluded that animal experiments were not the way to resolve any remaining doubts about Semmelweis's theory of the cause of child bed fever ("how childbed fever came into being") and that this could only be done by accumulating further clinical experience:

> Last autumn, at the request of Professor Skoda, this esteemed Section (*Classe*) asked me to conduct experiments in animals with Dr. Ignaz Semmelweis, in view of his statements about how puerperal fever came into being... Dr. Semmelweis had already in the spring and summer made these attempts with great zeal and conscientiousness, and carried out the post-mortems on the aniBrücke mals with me. These have, however,

---

[20] Murphy's translation of this portion of Semmelweis's *Aetiology* contains an error because he translated the original text '*und nach vollem Abschlusse verőffentlich werden sollen*' as '*and after complete analysi will be published*', which incorrectly suggested that the experiments had been completed when Haller wrote his full report. (SM, 565)

> until now delivered only ambiguous result, and have convinced me that experiments on animals are not the suitable means to lift the doubts about this important, and for everyone in whose eyes human life still has some value, interesting topic, rather, that this can only happen through the collection of experiences similar to those Dr. Semmelweis made in the local obstetrical institution in such a philanthropic way. (vGy, 288-289; Appendix B)

Semmelweis clearly took Brücke's conclusions about animal experiments to heart for he wrote in his *Aetiology*, after quoting Brucke's memorandum in its entirety:

> Since then [i.e. the experiments he had conducted with Brücke] I have had similar experiences as in Vienna in two other institutions;[21] I have also compiled in this text the similar experiences of others, and believe that as a result of the full impact of these experiences, experiments on animals are superfluous. (vGy, 289).

Lesky ignored all this: one could never have learned even of the existence of Brücke's memorandum from Lesky's monograph, or from her subsequent book about the Vienna Medical School. (Lesky, 187). Without knowing what Skoda had told the Academy of Sciences about Semmelweis's theory and the need for further animal experiments to resolve the doubts about it, it is impossible to understand why Semmelweis did not use his work on childbed fever as primary support for his application for *habilitation*.[22] Lesky made much of the fact that Semmelweis used primarily his essays on the modification of an obstetrical procedure for his *habilitation*-thesis, the novelty of which was

---

[21] This is a reference to Semmelweis's experiences in St. Rókus Hospital, where he reduced the frequency of childbed fever to 0.85% by implementing chlorine hand-disinfection, and to the results he obtained at the university hospital after being appointed Professor of Obstetrics at the University of Pest in July, 1855, where he reduced the maternal mortality rate from childbed fever to 0.39% after implementing chlorine hand-disinfection. (SM, 413-416; S, 172).

[22] '*Habilitation*' is a higher examination a person must pass to be able to teach in a university and hold a professorship. It consists of a thesis based on original research, conducted independently—i.e. not supervised by an advisor—which the candidate then has to defend before a committee.

open to question, and relegated his work on childbed fever to a subsidiary role. [**M, 65**] However, Semmelweis's reluctance to use his research on childbed fever as the main thesis becomes readily understandable once one understands that Semmelweis's account of his discovery would have been inconsistent with the account Skoda had given to the Academy of Sciences, since Skoda did not give a correct account of Semmelweis's discovery, and Semmelweis himself alluded to this in his *Aetiology*:

> Scanzoni...has not even been able to learn the true cause of childbed fever from Skoda's discourse, who had indeed mentioned some things not pertaining to childbed fever. (SM, 619)

Once it is also realized that far from tracing the logical steps that led Semmelweis to his discovery, Skoda repeatedly said that doubts remained about Semmelweis's theory whenever Skoda spoke about it in public, Semmelweis's reluctance to publish his work in Vienna until leaders of the Vienna Medical School and scientific community felt those doubts had been resolved also becomes readily understandable. But it was Skoda himself who had made it impossible for Semmelweis to resolve those doubts in Vienna, not the speculative psychological problem to which Lesky attributed Semmelweis's failure to publish his research earlier.

Skoda first told the College of Professors that the results of the chlorine hand-disinfection experiment left doubts about the correctness of Semelweis's theory of the cause of childbed fever. Next, he told the Academy of Sciences that the animal experiments Semmelweis had conducted to resolve those doubts had failed to resolve them, and that Semmelweis needed to conduct further and more varied animal experiments to resolve those doubts. Semmelweis conducted these additional experiments with the Brücke, but Brücke concluded that the only way to resolve the doubts about the cause of childbed fever was through further clinical observations, not animal experiments. However, by causing Klein not to renew his Assistantship, Skoda had deprived Semmelweis of the ability to accumulate the evidence Brücke said was necessary to resolve the very doubts Skoda repeatedly spoke about in public. (vGy, 36, 40, 45; Appendix A, pp. 161, 167, 172-173)

Once account is taken of all that Lesky omitted from her narrative the question turns to Skoda's motivation: onto why, as Lesky put it, 'Skoda adopted Semmelweis's discovery in a way as if it was his own business.' [**M, 57**]. Were the devastating consequences that Skoda's involvement in Semmelweis's research had on Semmelweis and his theory simply the unintended consequences of a well-intentioned but obtuse man, or were they calculated to arrogate to Skoda and the Vienna Medical School credit for Semmelweis's discovery at a time when Vienna was trying to replace Paris as the capital of the medical world? After all, Lesky herself conceded that if Semmelweis's inferences were not somehow linked intellectually to Skoda and the Vienna Medical School 'it was only given to this school to connect anatomically established facts with findings in the living, and to evaluate them diagnostically.' [**M, 57**]

Exactly so. Skoda became a brilliant diagnostician, whose lasting contributions to the diagnosis of cardiac and chest diseases made him famous throughout Europe,[23] but his contributions were made by applying techniques and ideas that were not his own, but those of others who were not members of the Vienna Medical School: Auenbrugger's technique of percussion, (FG, 354-355), Laennec's technique of auscultation, (FG, 411-412), and the idea of correlating clinical signs and symptoms of disease with autopsy findings that originated with Morgagni in Padua, was developed by Baillie in England, and Bichat and others in Paris, and eventually extended by Rokitansky (see below). Lesky's claim about Semmelweis's discovery being made with methods he learned from others was true of Skoda, not Semmelweis; in this respect, Skoda may be said to have been Salieri to Semmelweis's Mozart.

It is true that half a dozen or so of the faculty of the Vienna Medical School and AKH supported and spoke up for Semmelweis, but they were never able to circumvent the dead hand of bureaucracy on education. Even after the old regulations were relaxed and Rokitansky became the first freely elected Dean of the Medical School on October 1, 1849, [**M, 55**], he was unable to secure for Semmelweis a position as

[23] Sakula.

Privatdozent (docent)[24] that would have allowed Semmelweis to practice clinical obstetrics, give demonstrations on cadavers, and issue students who had enrolled in his course on obstetrics certificates of attendance and satisfactory completion. The position of docent to which he was named on October 1, 1850 limited Semmelweis only to "demonstrating and practicing on manikins," so he left Vienna, and later explained that he did because

> Such a limited docentur would be of no benefit to me, since the statute requires just as broad an instruction on the part of the decent as the Professor for certification by the docent to be valid, but it was permissible for the Professor to give demonstrations and exercises on the cadaver. (SM, 413)

But Lesky insisted that Semmelweis's appointment as docent 'was the first tangible success in the great struggle that the Rokitansky-Skoda School had achieved in their nearly two-year tough struggle for Semmelweis,' and that Semmelweis's incomprehensible departure from Vienna was likely the result of a psychological problem:

> If one combines all these facts in the newly discovered documents with Semmelweis's attempt to justify his sudden departure from Vienna...with the restriction on his docenture, one cannot but help diagnose that this attempt represents a later self-interpretation. Here Semmelweis's case stops being historical and starts to become more psychological. [**M. 78**]

Lesky acknowledged that Semmelweis had correctly interpreted the decree 'on the position, duties and rights of private docents in educational institutions' as precluding him from issuing certificates of attendance and satisfactory completion to students who had elected to take his course on obstetrics, but she accused Semmelweis of being disingenuous because

> This decree was issued on January 5, 1849, and Semmelweis must have known about it long before May 9, 1850, when he

---

[24] '*Privatdozent*' is a title, not a salaried position, conferred by European universities on someone who is qualified and permitted to teach a certain subject at a university.

expressed his readiness to restrict his lectures to demonstration on phantoms. [**M, 78**]

But Lesky's argument again ignored facts. It is true that when Semmelweis was notified that his appointment limited him to demonstrations on phantoms, he had already accepted the restriction when he applied for the position on May 9, 1850; and it is also true that he knew that the restriction would not allow him to issue certificates of satisfactory attendance and completion to students as this was made clear in a decree on January 5, 1849. But it is equally true that Semmelweis's willingness to limit his demonstrations to manikins ("phantoms") was only '*until the cadaver-question is definitively settled by the* High Ministry,' i.e. provisional, [**M-70**], and it was not unreasonable for Semmelweis to have supposed that the question would be settled before his renewed application for a docentur was decided, and decided in his favor, given that Rokitansky was now Dean and supported the use of cadavers for teaching by docents. [**M, 72-73**] Obviously, this expectation was dashed, and after reconsidering all that the restrictions on his appointment implied, Semmelweis decided to leave Vienna. Lesky deemed this 'incomprehensible' because 'the possibility of extending the limited docenture already loomed.' [**M, 77**] However, Lesky never justified her conclusory speculation, nor confirmed that the possibility she contended "loomed" was ever actually realized—i.e. she never showed, either in her monograph or subsequent book on the Vienna Medical School, that the regulations were subsequently amended to permit docents to use cadavers for teaching and demonstrations.

In the final section of her monograph, Lesky chronicled the appointment of Klein's successor following Klein's death in April, 1856, and made—although not quite expressly—the kind of counterfactual claim that history can never warrant: that were it not for the fact that Semmelweis had not published 'a single line in nine years,' he would have been appointed to succeed Klein as professor in Vienna. **[M-92, 93]**. It was the natural apogee of Lesky's attempt to place responsibility for Semmelweis's professional fate in Vienna solely on Semmelweis himself.

Lesky set the stage for this claim in the preceding section of her monograph in which she described Semmelweis's appointment to replace

Johann Birly, professor of obstetrics at the University of Pest, who had been one of Klein's assistants, and who had died on November 25, 1854. Lesky noted 'with all soberness that even Semmelweis's home was not at first ready to offer the country's greatest son the positon which his achievement should have secured him.' **[M-78]** This was all the more remarkable, Lesky said, given that there was a requirement that individuals appointed to professorship within the Habsburg lands speak the native language of the country in which they were appointed, and Carl Braun, the Pest faculty's first choice, did not speak Hungarian. Lesky concluded that the only reason Semmelweis was not the faculty's preferred choice was that Braun had co-authored a textbook on obstetrics that had received critical acclaim both at home and abroad, whereas Semmelweis, as of 1855, 'had not written a line.' **[M-82]**

The appointment of Birly's replacement fell within the jurisdiction of the civil and military administration for Hungary in Vienna, and it sought the opinion of the Pest faculty. However, Benedek pointed out that the Pest faculty was not familiar with the details of obstetrical practice—Semmelweis's long-time friend Lajos Markusovszky was not a member of the Pest faculty—and the faculty's choice was limited to Carl Braun, Semmelweis, and Birly's former assistant, Frank Walla, who was 'as undistinguished and backward-looking as his chief had been.' (B, 170) Benedek also pointed out that the professors on the Pest faculty were also very average, and if they knew anything at all about Semmelweis's discovery, they likely knew only that his views were controversial. In addition, the professors were loyalists who had supported the monarchy during Hungary's war of independence, and while that did not excuse the national shame of not making Semmelweis their preferred choice, the faculty's choice was hardly inexplicable or surprising. (B, 170-171)

Lesky concluded her account of Semmelweis appointment in Pest by noting that Alexander von Helfert, the Undersecretary of State for Education, who had been outspoken in his opposition to the extension of Semmelweis's assistantship in 1849, now gave a glowing account of Semmelweis's research in his request to the Emperor to appoint Semmelweis professor in Pest. Lesky inferred from this that during the

Thun-Hohenstein era 'a drastic change had occurred towards Semmelweis within Austria's highest authority.' She drew this inference and her conclusion about why Semmelweis had not been the Pest faculty's first choice to bolster her final grand conclusion that Semmelweis in fact enjoyed so much support from the progressive members of the Vienna Medical School that had it not been for the fact that 'Semmelweis could not bring himself to publish the slightest amount until 1857,' Semmelweis would have been appointed to replace Klein as professor on the first maternity clinic.

Klein died in April, 1856. Semmelweis had not applied for his post but the Appointments Committee (*Besetzungskomitee*) solicited applications from physicians both inside and outside Austria, including Semmelweis. [**M, 84-85**] Schürer von Waldheim had concluded that the reason Semmelweis was not appointed to succeed Klein was that he had rejected the docentur he was granted and abruptly left Vienna, and 'one does not want to expose oneself to such treatment a second time,' but Lesky poured cold water on Schürer's conclusion. She noted that the Appointments Committee laid special emphasis on the literary achievements of applicants, and concluded that the only reason Semmelweis was not appointed to succeed Klein was because 'Semmelweis had not a single line...on any subject in his field:'

> As far as the additional qualification and teaching ability are concerned, the committee finds itself prompted here to mention in particular Professor Semmelweis, who... received full approval and support from many thoughtful investigators for his view of the origin of puerperal diseases...; however, recognizing this merit, the members of the committee must all the more regret that Professor Semmelweis has not published in his field during these last few years, which literary works it would have like to point to, and to have seen follow his otherwise eminent skills. [**M, 85-86**]

However, after assuming his position as professor in Pest and implementing chlorine hand-disinfection the previous year, Semmelweis lost only 2 of 514 (0.39%) mothers to childbed fever during his first eleven months in the post, and Semmelweis's assistant. József Fleischer, reported the results in the Vienna Medical Weekly (*Wiener Medizinische Wochenschrift*), only to receive the following derisory Editorial Comment:

> We thought this theory of chlorine disinfection had died out long ago: the experience and statistical evidence of most of the lying-in institutions protest against the opinions expressed in this article: it would be well that our readers should not allow themselves to be misled by this theory at the present time. (S,127)

Lesky acknowledged but discounted the article as irrelevant because the Appointments Committee had already acknowledged that Semmelweis's doctrine had "received full approval and support from many thoughtful investigators," and Fleischer's report could add nothing to those conclusions. But this is to miss the point. What is relevant is not Fleischer's report but the editorial response to the report for it contradicts the statements in the Appointments Committee's report about the approval that Semmelweis's theory had ostensibly received from many thoughtful investigators. It is difficult to believe that the Appointments Committee would not have been aware of the opposition that Semmelweis's theory continued to face in Vienna as Franz Bartsch, professor on the second maternity division, who had also been one of Klein's assistants and who also rejected Semmelweis's theory, was a member of the Appointments Committee, [**M-84**], and this in turn casts doubt on whether the stated reasons for not appointing Semmelweis were the actual reasons. Indeed, Semmelweis was offered the chair of obstetrics in Zurich notwithstanding that he had still not published his *Aetiology*, (G-Z, 100-101), which is inconsistent with the dispositive influence that Lesky attributed to Semmelweis's lack of publications. Semmelweis had substantive reasons for not publishing his work sooner, as discussed in the critique of Lesky's historical narrative.

SEMMELWEIS AND THE VIENNA MEDICAL SCHOOL

ERNA LESKY

[7] Introduction

The years 1847-1850 are associated with one of the greatest discoveries in the history of medicine, and were the decisive ones in Semmelweis's life. Although accounts of it still remained connected to Viennese soil and the Vienna Medical School, it is surprising how little new data and historical analysis have been added to the biographies of Semmelweis written in the nineteenth and early twentieth century to clarify the important phases of that discovery. Essentially one had to be content with Fritz Schürer von Waldheim's biography. Schürer tried to collect the widely scattered literature on Semmelweis's doctrine, and it may have been commendable for his day notwithstanding the deficiencies in his use of the archival materials in the Ministry of Education and University Archives, 'but his frequent use of 'probably,' 'perhaps,' and 'possibly' should have alerted any astute historian to how tentative his conclusions were.'

Never the less, the incomplete, hypothetical picture **[8]** that Schürer painted of Semmelweis's Vienna years, and all the difficulties associated with his discovery, were accepted uncritically as what research on Semmelweis had established despite the fact that Schürer had conflated what was merely hypothetical with what had been established as veridical ("attested to") in a very confusing way. And this picture has been perpetuated, without contradiction, not only in the German, but also in the Anglo-Saxon literature on Semmelweis by the work of Sir William Sinclair, which appeared four years after Schürer's biography; Sinclair followed Schürer entirely, although he did clarify Semmelweis's priority over the Anglo-American contagionists.

The accepted view of this history was actually based on *assumed* historical facts and simplified what in reality was the playing out of a very complex power struggle into a personal conflict between a backward professor and his forward-looking, ingenious assistant. It was accepted that Semmelweis's chief and professor of Obstetrics in Vienna, Johann Klein, and his influential backers, were Semmelweis's opponents, but in reality Klein and Semmelweis **[9]** were involved in a conflict of far greater dimension, the context of which had an extraordinarily complicated administrative and educational historical background. 'The main actors in this struggle were Joseph Skoda, the pioneer of a new medicine based on exact scientific methods, and Anton von Rosas, a Hungarian-born ophthalmologist, and a yesterday's man, who was provisional vice-director of medical education between 1848 and 1850.'

[11] Anton von Rosas and Jonathan Klein

Lesky prefixed her brief description of Klein and Rosas's professional careers with a short summary of the Austrian authoritarian educational system that had its genesis in the absolutist era of the Habsburg monarchy in the eighteenth century that began with the accession of Maria Theresa as Empress in 1740.

The highest central teaching authority was the Court Study Commission. Maria Theresa's personal physician, Gerard van Swieten, a Dutchman, created the post of Director of Medical Studies which was linked to the work of the Court Study Commission while van Swieten and his successor, Anton von Störck, occupied the post: van Swieten acted as the Commission's vice president, and Störck was an associate member.

'Leopold II dissolved both the Court Study Commission and the study directorate in 1790 as an experiment in the self-administration of universities. But when the principle of authoritative paternalism was restored under Franz I,[25] the study directorate was the first to be restored

[25] Francis I (1768-1835) became Emperor Francis II of the Habsburg Empire on the sudden death of Leopold II in 1792. He was also the last Holy Roman Emperor, as the Holy Roman Empire ceased to exist after 1806.

at the instigation of his personal physician, Joseph Andreas von Stifft (1760-1836) in 1802, followed by the Court Study Commission in 1808, and from then on Stifft served as an associate on the Commission. However, under established administrative practices, the same person could not occupy these two offices at the same time, so in 1811 the office of Vice-director of Medical Studies of the University of Vienna was created; the vice-director had to deal with all teaching-related matters, report to the Director of Medical Studies on all important matters, and be bound by his decision.'

At the time that the absolutist Austrian state was exerting its authority over higher education through these offices, as restored and modified by Stifft, other German-speaking countries were moving in the opposite direction: toward autonomy in university constitutions. However, in Vienna 'it was still the task of the vice-director to see that instructors followed the prescribed textbooks to the letter; for they were not authorized to depart from the principles laid down in them, much less substitute others, or their own notebooks, for the prescribed textbooks [and] it was also part of the official duties of the vice-director often to attend lectures unexpectedly, and observe the lectures of the professors, and, at the same time, the behavior and progress of the students at college exams. Assistants like Semmelweis, no less than professors, were also under the supervision of the vice-director, and their official duties were governed by the detailed instructions of March 31, 1818.'

'All these instructions, which were still fully in force during Semmelweis's assistantship, came mostly from Stifft's office, and were significantly eased after Stifft's death, when Ludwig Freiherr von Turkheim came to prominence. Türkheim was a student of Johann Peter Frank, and by 1811 had already held the office of vice-director of medical studies, which he then resigned to take over the post of medical officer at the court chancellery. He had a significant influence on the organization of medical education when he became an assessor on the Court Study Commission, as from this position Turkheim guided the young talent of the second Viennese Medical School, and set a course very different from the bureaucratic despotism of the Stifft era, even before it was legally eliminated by the reforms of the Minister of Education, Leo Grafen Thun-

Hohenstein in 1849. So it is understandable that in his inaugural lecture in 1846, Skoda described Türkhei as "a second van Swieten," who "did not lag behind, but for years worked to reform medical studies in Austria, and whose execution was hindered only by his death."'

'The disastrous consequences for the young faculty of the death of this far-sighted and generous man in 1846, one year before Semmelweis's epoch-making discovery, were not immediately apparent because Türkheim was at first succeeded by Ernst von Feutersleben, who shared Türkheim's reform-minded leadership. Only after Feuchtersleben resigned both as undersecretary of the newly-created Ministry of Education as well as vice-director of medical studies in the revolutionary year of 1848 that the full extent of the disaster became apparent. And it was a grotesque irony that Anton von Rosas, who was the sworn enemy of everything new, and thereby Skoda's natural enemy, and under whose vice-directorship the group reformers around Skoda and Rokitansky saw their hopes, which they had set on the year 1848, dashed should have been nominated to replace Feuchtersleben as vice-director of medical studies on December 23, 1848 by none other than Skoda himself.

Rosas and Klein graduated doctors of medicine in the same year (1816), they were both employed as second assistants at the *Allgemeines Krankenhaus* in the same year (1818), and were also first assistants at the same time. Both were just 30 years old when they were named professors, Klein in Salzburg and Rosas in Padua. Anyone who became a professor at such a young age had to be in favor with the all-powerful director of medical studies, Joseph Andreas von Stifft, and to be considered by him to have had the right attitude and way of thinking. Klein and Rosas fitted what Stifft wanted in a professor so well that they both returned within a short period of time to Vienna and to professorships with a European reputation. In 1821, Rosas took over the eye clinic from George Joseph Beers, considered the leader in his field, and in the following year Klein took over from Johann Lukas Boer, who had acquired a European reputation as the founder of natural midwifery. Klein maintained that reputation for 34 years, but only because his department became the 'breeding ground of puerperal fever.' 'During his 34 years as head of the then largest obstetrical clinic in the world, Klein exhausted his dutires by being a conscientious book-keeper of childbed fever, and, through his annual reports, an exact registrant of each *genius epidemicus* that gave rise to this fever.'

Rosas was different. He was an excellent teacher and surgeon, which Klein was not. He also compiled a useful textbook, which the critics approved. But, most importantly, he became more well versed in Austrian university regulations and practices than any member of the faculty through his compilation and diligent study of the files and older statues of the Viennese Medical School, and which he published in 1847. Rosas combined legal expertise with literary sophistication as the editor of the Medical Yearbook of the Imperial State Government, which he edited with Stifft's son-in-law until 1841, whereafter he became the main editor. His evil bent became evident in 1842, when he published an article, "On the Sources of Today's Medical Misbehavior and the Means of Controlling it Effectively." 'When he also attacked Jewish doctors and others in this article, it was clear that, with Rosas, Stifft's stamp of conservatism had found not only a very aggressive, but a dangerously intolerant representative.'

On December 30, 1848, Rosas was entrusted with the management of the medical College of Professors. It was a time when the educational reforms announced in March 1848, although not yet codified, left little doubt that they would secure to the academic authorities the right of self-administration. However, instead of paving the way for the reform of higher education that was enacted with Thun's Higher Eductional Organization Act of 30 September, 1849, Rosas opposed these developments under the university regulations that still remained in force 'with intolerant zeal.'

One object in this struggle has been the recognition and enforcement of Semmelweis's discovery. 'When the group of reformers around Skoda and Rokitansky fought for them with all the means at their disposal, Semmelweis's cause became almost a **[17]** test case for whether the self-government which had been granted to the faculty would actually be allowed. The fundamental meaning of Semmelweis's case in the framework of the university reform of 1848 has been overlooked so far. To understand it, it is necessary clearly to define the basic legal position from which the reformers group around Skoda and Rokitansky, i.e. the second Viennese school, took up its fight for Semmelweis.'

On March 12, 1848, when the Vienna riots began, the students and faculty demanded freedom of teaching and learning in their petition to the Emperor and their demands were granted in the imperial patent of March 15, 1848, and set forth in the decree of April 6, the most important provisions were the following:

> The immediate direction of each individual educational institution, both at the so-called four faculty studies, as well as all technical institutes and all grammar schools, is hereby conferred on the faculty of the same, which is made up of the members of each such study department; that is, the vice-director or grammar-school prefect as chairman, and all the actual professors of the same as leaders in a college, to undertake the custody and decision of all those study matters, by joint decision after the results of the majority vote, which according to the previous regulations could be decided for them locally or by the state office of the province…
>
> By broadening the scope of the faculty, and entrusting the management of higher studies directly to men of science themselves, the Ministry is expressing its confidence that they will also carry out this important charge in the spirit of true scientific development, and with their insight and experience, the Ministry of Education will eagerly support sincere pursuits in all directions to give our fatherland's teaching institutions a lively upturn.
>
> The foundations on which the teaching staff must operate [**18**] until new instructions for all branches of public educational instructions are given by legislation in a constitutional manner, are the existing legal provisions that remain in force insofar as they do not appear to be repealed by the above orders.
>
> Nonetheless, wherever the Ministry of Education declares it to be desirable to abolish any existing institution or provision, even before the desirability of a new study legislation is definitely established, it will endeavor temporarily to lift such infirmities for the time being.

'Because of the interim character of this decree, there were no separate instructions for the provisional vice-director, and it depended solely on his discretion to what extent he was willing faithfully to interpret the wishes and decisions of the faculty.'

Skoda's application for the appointment of an inquiry commission

On July 19, 1848 Feuchtersleben left the post of vice-director of medical studies and became Undersecretary in the Ministry of Education; Joseph Wattmann (1789-1866), a surgeon and the senior member of the faculty, became vice-director and his deputy was Casper Fisher, professor of natural history. 'As far as one could tell from the minutes of the medical College of Professors, there were no conflicts during Wattmann's time in the post even though the College of Professors, like the university, was heavily burdened.'

A ministerial decree ensured that Feuchtersleben could return to his post as vice-director 'in the event of a change in ministerial relations,' and Feuchtersleben relied on this decree to return to the vice-directorate on December 14, 1848 after he resigned as undersecretary. The cause of Feuchtersleben's resignation was the order he issued in October, 1848 to dismiss five professors on the medical faculty, which Skoda put into effect on December 23, 1848. The Ministry of Education censured the College of Medical Professors for this action at a meeting on January 16, 1849 stating that the College had exceeded the scope of its authority. Feuchtersleben was replaced as Undersecretary of Education by Alexander von Helfert (1820-1910), who complained about the medical faculty's rekindling of the anti-government rivalry that had prevailed since 'premodern times,' and 'aggravated the hostile attitude of the Ministry towards the medical faculty, which had only increased since the events in October.'

Classes at the university had ended on May, 24, 1848, and the university buildings from which the March revolution had begun remained a barracks so that not only could lectures not **[19]** begin in the autumn of 1848, 'but the October Revolution also brought new turmoil and a state of emergency in the city after its suppression [and] it was not until the end of the year, as the situation slowly began to normalize, that it was possible to think of resuming the program of studies.' And 'the time had also come to deal with the discovery in the medical College of Professors that the Assistant on the 1st maternity clinic, Semmelweis, had made in May 1847, and that for 1½ years now had proved so successful. Yes, it had to be done, since this assistant's request to extend his service by two years was submitted on December 1, 1848. However, this could not be settled in Wattann's time, because the deadline for applications for this position, 20th December, had to be waited out. As we know from the later reports of Klein and Bartsch, Semmelweis referred in his application to the fact that only extension of his service would give him the opportunity to prove without any doubt the success of the previous chlorine washings.'

'The same desire to break new paths of discovery drove the man who subsequently proved to be Semmelweis's energetic champion, Joseph Skoda. Therefore, at the meeting on January 16, 1849, he moved for the formation of a commission to examine the cause of the different mortality rates at the first and second maternity divisions. Thus, two matters involving Semmelweis came up for discussion at the beginning of 1849: the request for an extension, and Skoda's motion. Even though these were two different official processes, as things stood, the one, Skoda's application, could not but have a retroactive effect on the other, Semelweis's petition. Besides, Skoda, Semmelweis's lawyer [*Amwalt*], had at the same time made himself the spokesman for the reform group on important issues [**20**] directly affecting university reform—such as membership of the Colleges, especially regarding exceptional professors and lecturers; the question of the *habilitation* standards and the prospective curriculum—all pressing issues requiring decision, but that were nevertheless likely to involve the movant in a plethora of conflicts with the vice-director on the one hand, and entangle it with the Ministry on the other.'

It was in this tense atmosphere, compounded by Feuchterslebens's removal, and the Ministry's censure of the College in which Skoda was embroiled, that Skoda made his motion concerning Semmelweis's discovery, and which was presided over by Rosas. 'Schürer von Waldheim had created confusion by reprinting not the text of the original motion but the academic lecture Skoda gave nine months later on 18 October 1849.' The text of the minutes of January 16, 1849 was as follows:

[21] 16. Finally, Prof. Skoda made the following motion:

'Over many years, the mortality rate on the first maternity clinic exceeded that on the second clinic. In the month of June, 1847, the number of deaths suddenly fell, and remained low for the rest of the year. From January 1 until the end of May, of 1534 women giving birth, 120 died. From June 1, 1847 to the end of December, 1847, only 56 of 1841 women giving birth died.

In 1848, this ratio exceeding all expectations; out of 3556 deliveries, only 45 died. In earlier years, the mortality ratio was constant and enormous:

1840 : 2810 Giving Birth	267 Died
1841 : 2845	238
1842 : 3067	521
1843 : 2871	279
1844 : 2918	260
1845 : 3255	241
1846 : 3354	459

The College of Professors, being an association of men entrusted with the care of medical science, is obliged to deal with the cause of the previously great and now much reduced mortality, and to publish the results of the investigation. This obligation is still greater as it is the leading authority of medical studies. Prof. Skoda made the following request, that a Commission of 3-5 members of the faculty be selected without delay to investigate the relationship between the two maternity clinics, and to present the results of the investigation as soon as possible to the faculty.'

The following resolution is attached to Skoda's motion:

After a few remarks by Prof. Klein about the cause of that epidemic being still unidentified despite repeated medical inspections ordered by a higher authority, there was a unanimous vote to set up a three-member commission to act in the way Prof. Skoda had indicated. The majority of secret ballots were for Profs. Rokitansky, Shuh, and Skoda, who should deal immediately with the task mentioned.

'It can be seen that Skoda was insisting orally in this motion, as later in his written statement, that the decree of 6 April 1848 conferred on the faculty the right to act as the main authority of medical studies. Indeed, according to the text of the decree, "that (men of science) carry out this essential custody in a true spirit of scientific development," he considered it the faculty's duty to arrange for the exact scientific examination of a discovery already eagerly discussed in Kiel, Amsterdam and London. Thus, the Semmelweis matter necessarily became the touchstone of the good will of the supervisory authority to make the promised autonomy a reality.'

'But to understand the debate of Skoda's motion by the faculty it was necessary to correct an error that had been part of the Semmelweis literature since Schürer von Waldheim's time: namely, the claim that Skoda's motion was accepted "by a very large majority," which the minutes of the meeting revealed to be untrue. Rather, the faculty voted in two stages: first it voted on Skoda's motion for the appointment of an investigating commission, and second, it selected, by secret ballot, the members of the Commission. The text of the minutes show that Skoda's motion was not adopted "by a very large majority" but unanimously, which means that Klein also voted in favor of the motion and, in principle, agreed to the appointment of an investigating commission at this meeting. It was only after the members of the commission selected by secret ballot— Professors Rokistansky, Shuh and Skoda—did not include Klein that Klein's willingness to appoint a commission changed. As head of the clinic on which the Commission was supposed to take action, he may have hoped—and rightly so—that he himself would be chairman of this commission, or at least be a member.'

To point this out was not to condone Klein's later stance, but only to fulfill what an objective report requires: 'to describe accurately the exact actions that have set the course of an historical event. The effect of not nominating Klein a member of the commission became apparent four days later, when, at a meeting of January 20, Klein submitted his objection to the commission. The following is the text of his objection:'

> **[23]** I protest in the most solemn manner against the first decision of the teaching staff, namely:
>
> 1. Because the supposed scientific objective—to research an essentially unknown epidemic at a time and at a place where it does not exist—directly contradict sound principles of human reason, and because of that cannot be truly scientific;
>
> 2. Because a member of the College, Professor Skoda, has himself proved that he is my personal enemy, as anyone can take away from his recent remarks;
>
> 3. Because under the Ministry's provision of December 18 of last year, the College itself is not entitled to interfere with a professor, who has for many years rendered honorable service, in a way that is capable of undermining his honor;
>
> 4. Because my accuser is among the commission entrusted with the investigation, indeed, a new selection is also likely to fall on his close friends, from whom, therefore, an impartial investigation and a fair judgment cannot be expected.
>
> I don't shy away from any investigating commission, I have no reason to, there have already been several at different times when the epidemic struck, and remained at a higher level; but I demand a commission of non-partisan experts, who alone are appropriate to express a well-grounded opinion, and who are called only for this purpose.
>
> And should the faculty persist with its decision, I am resolved to appeal to the wisdom and justice of the Ministry of Education, and until a decision follows from on high, I solemnly forbid in the appropriate sense each procedure the faculty might undertake.
>
> *Vienna, 20th January, 1849* — *Dr J. Klein*
> *Prof. Der 1ten geburtshilflichen Klinik*

The text of these arguments reveals that Klein's objections were purely personal in that he described Skoda as his 'accuser' and 'personal enemy,' and his honor as professor and head of the clinic wounded. But it was only because of the incompleteness of the source materials that Schürer of Waldheim used that the Klein: Skoda: Semmelweis altercation had been branded as a purely personal dispute, and if one followed the Semmelweis case systematically based on the minutes of the proceedings, a very different and substantively deeper aspect became apparent.

'The discussion had already turned to this more fundamental principle on February 3, when Klein's objection was debated at Skoda's request. The botanist, Stephan Endlicher (1804-184), who opposed the appointment of an investigating commission, raised the novel and momentous argument that the appointment of such a commission of inquiry exceeds the faculty's authority. In doing so, Endlicher—preceded one may presume by a consultation with Rosas—elevated what had previously been construed as a purely personal dispute into a fundamental debate on the most burning issue of those years: 'the realization of the university's autonomy from the Ministry of Education.'

'Skoda opposed Endlicher's view at that meeting, and at the subsequent meeting on February 10, submitted a justification of his position in writing that is of central historical importance to the Semmelweis case, but that has been overlooked by previous Semmelweis research. By publishing it here for the first time, we believe that we have wrested at one and the same time one of the most beautiful testimonies of the real spirit of research and grand artistry from the dustbin of the archives. For in this document Skoda does not content himself with justifying the legality of his proposal for the supervision of investigations granted to the faculty in the decree of April 6, 1848; it is characteristic of Skoda's elevated concept of his role as researcher and teacher that he regards this right as a self-evident duty steeped in the faculty's scholarly mission, and thus deduced it from areas beyond injunctions and ordinances. In recognizing it as a duty of "every teacher as well as the faculty as a whole" to deal with the solution of medical problems, he located the Semmelweiss question, the clarification of the causes of puerperal fever, in that ideal space of duty in which the doctor feels ultimately responsible only for the suffering of mankind. The text of this vote is:'

[25] I. Supplement to Protocol for February 10, 1849:

Justification for the faculty's majority vote at the meeting on February 3 regarding the faculty's authority to form a commission with the aim of investigating the causes of the mortality rate at the 1st maternity clinic, which in earlier years had been enormous but for a year and a half had been significantly reduced.

That the unanimous decision of the faculty on 16 January to form a commission to determine the causes of the mortality on the 1st obstetric clinic, which had been so enormous but suddenly reduced for a year and a half, came up for debate on February 3 following the protest tabled by Prof. Klein on 20 January, and the minority of the faculty expressed the view that the faculty was not authorized to form such a commission, and thus exceeded the scope of its authority by the decision it took on January 16.

From the following considerations, it should be apparent that this minority view is untenable:

The expansion of medical knowledge is the responsibility of each individual member of the faculty just as it is of the faculty collectively. Accordingly, it is not only the medical faculty's right, but obligation to the State and humanity, to concern itself with solving medical questions.

But if the faculty has a duty to the state and humanity to expand medical knowledge, it must have the right to deal with the solution of medical problems even against the wishes of individual members. Therefore, this right, as a necessary consequence of the duty of the faculty, cannot be denied even if it was not appointed the governing authority. Under the present circumstances, when it has been entrusted with the supervision of individual Professors and their institutions, the faculty would be stamped by public opinion as neglecting its responsibility, if under important occasions it did want to exercise this right. Could there be a more important occasion on which to exercise this right than the present case!

The fact that until June, 1847, the mortality on the first clinic was permanently and significantly higher than on the second clinic, is still a very important medical question.

This fact had for a long time been of concern to physicians in home and foreign countries, and to the whole Viennese public, and forced the authorities repeatedly to discuss it in committees, which, however, had no result, since the mortality remained the same as before.

Since June, 1847, the mortality dropped strikingly, indeed, was less than on the second clinic. As far as we know, nothing changed in the relationship between the clinics, only that Dr. Semmelweis, the assistant, ordered that no one was allowed to examine laboring women without first cleaning their hands in chlorine water. He made this provision on the supposition that because loose rotting organic matter contaminated the hands of students if they were employed in the autopsy room, women in labor perhaps become infected, and this brings about childbed fever.

Dr. Semmelweis came to this supposition after carefully comparing the circumstances of the two clinics; it turned out that among pregnant and laboring women, there were, neither in the medical nor dietary treatments, nor in the findings on examination, any differences between the two clinics, and also that the midwives never dealt with autopsies, and so never contaminated their hands with loose organic matter, but this kind of soiling occurred frequently among the students. The fact that the disease also occurred on the second maternity clinic could not be used as an objection to this supposition, as for the time being this was not treated as an issue about clarifying all the causes of childbed fever, but merely about finding out and preventing the root cause of the disproportionately high mortality rate on the first maternity clinic.

As much as now the experience of one and a half years seems to confirm the presumption of Dr. Semmelweis, as surprising as the success achieved in Kiel through Semmelweis's method of chlorinewashing is, that matter has still not yet been clarified. The faculty can no longer be allowed to be an idle spectator, if what is at issue is that in one of the institutions entrusted to its supervision a discovery is made which, if proven, will belong to the most fruitful and useful discoveries in medical science. With such negligence the College would not only show its indifference to scientific endeavors, but its failure to assess and disclose such an important discovery would saddle the committee with responsibility for endangering the lives of many people.

10th February, 1849	*Jos. Skoda*
Dr. J. A. Raimann	*Prof. der med. Klinik*
Prof. der med. Klinik	*Carl Rokitansky*
Dr. Sigmund	*Prof. der path Anatomie*
Dr. Dumreicher	*Joh. Dlauthy*
Dr. Kainzbauer	*Prof. der Staatsarzneikunde*

The last sentence of this statement shows that Skoda, with all the keenness of his understanding, was not only aware of the significance of Semmelweis's discovery, but also felt deeply about it. For he saw in it, not only the control of a disease, but an example of the goal of his therapeutic endeavours: not as the old school did by prescribing recipes for the symptoms of diseases, but by understanding the disease itself, and still more, by preventing it from arising. It was on this casual reference to treatment, out of everything, that Ferdinand von Arlt called Skoda a "doctor in the grand style." The document presented here is alone sufficient to refute the criticism of Skoda's therapeutic nihilism, lodged against him by his contemporaries, and repeated over and over again since then.

'Never the less, one should not overlook that the logic of this vote implies that the faculty has a right to intervene in each individual member's activities, an interpretation of autonomy that necessarily led to serious conflicts. Here, it is important bring the right balance instead of an all too one-sided approach to Semmelweis's research and realize that the struggle for the recognition of Semmelweis's discovery crosses over into a problem that lies entirely different plane. The autonomy of an institute or clinic is today, as ever, a particularly delicate issue in the life of every university. It was brought up for debate by the failure to include clinical director Klein on the commission in a manner that threatened to jeopardize the entire question of autonomy. This is clearly shown by Klein's second protests on February 10, 1849, which also reprinted here for the first time:'

[28] II. Supplement to Protokoll of 10 February d. J. Z. VII N. 31.

The grounds for the view expressed by the undersigned and some of his colleagues on the 3rd of February, that the faculty's decision on January 16th to establish a commission to investigate the causes of the epidemic in the maternity clinic was not authorized, and thus by this decision had exceeded the scope of its activity:

As long as the organization of the faculty is provisional and the scope of its activities is not decided, the management of student affairs must be according to the old regulations, and insofar as the ordering of commission negotiations has so far only been carried out by the authorities, the faculty does not have the right to decide and initiate such a commission without authorization.

Furthermore, according to Professor Skoda's claim, to extend medical knowledge is the task and duty of every teacher as well as of the faculty as a whole; thus every single professor, not only the faculty as a whole, has the right to be able to deal with the solution of medical problems unhindered, and to reject any interference that he has recognized as being inappropriate and disruptive. As a result, even from this point of view, the faculty is not empowered with respect to its individual members, to appoint such a commission against the wishes of the individual, thereby impairing the individual's right to solve medical problems without interference.

After the epidemic of childbed fever ceased in the year 1847, the undersigned introduced chlorine washings on his clinic on the recommendation of his assistant. His assistant, who was clearly not authorized to introduce the washings himself, believed that childbed fever was caused by the transfer of loose organic matter to laboring women, and that washing the hands of students with chlorine instead of soap as earlier would remove the cause and with it the childbed fever epidemic. The undersigned considered the matter a scientific question that he, as Professor, not only had the right but the obligation to investigate. But the matter—as Professor Skoda has himself agreed—remained unclear, and had by no means been decided; yet, Professor Skoda has proposed, and a majority of the committee has approved, that a panel be appointed to evaluate the discovery and publicize it without delay, all because the latest epidemic had abated, since when hand disinfection with chlorine was implemented, and mortality greatly decreased.

Quite apart from being inconsistent, and a muddled and detrimental way to resolve the question, such a proposal and determination must be rejected, and this committee reported not only for being unauthorized to appoint such a panel, but all the more because, Professor Skoda's pretextual scientific intentions aside, the proposal couples the panel's self-interest with a hateful, inquisitional coloration; and because Professor Skoda is not hurrying to evaluate and disclose this as yet unrealized discovery for the sake of science or mankind, but in the interest of his followers before their support ends, and to the extent that a research subject matter is imaginable at all, surely nothing of any real value to science or mankind can be derived from the publication of a discovery not yet made.

Vienna 9th March, 1849

Dr. J. Klein
Prof. der geburtshilfe
Dr. Stephan Endlicher
k. k. Professor
K.D. Schroff
k. k. Professor
Rosas kk Prof
Dr. Seligmann
a. o. Professor

Dr. Bartsch
k. k. Professor
Prof. Schuh

'The significant of this document for the pre-March intellectual climate can be viewed from several angles. One can take it as a self-portrait of Klein; one can stress the new insight it provides for the development of Semmelweis's doctrine. We will do this later. But for now, we want to raise and consider the rights of the faculty [*fakultätsrechtlichen Betrachtung*]: Klein took full advantage of Endlicher's argument and, relying on the current provisional nature of the university constitution, denied the right of the faculty to form a commission. At the same time, Klein himself, and his legally expert aid [i.e. Rosas], relied on the same decree of April 6, 1848 that Skoda himself took as the legal basis for his motion. For nothing in this decree stipulated "the basis for the faculty to exercise its authority"... in other words, until new orders were provided in a constitutional manner by legislation for all branches of public education "the existing regulations are to remain." According to these, however, the appointment of the commissions was, since Stifft's time, assigned to the director of studies. These divergent interpretations reflected the ambivalence of this transitional decree that was so dangerous in Semmelweis's case. Klein and his sympathizers appealed to the old, but still existing regulations as the basis for rejecting the Commission, but had no qualms about relying on the new regulations that the faculty and each of its members had the right, indeed, the duty to free, unimpeded research, and thereby to turn Skoda's own arguments against Skoda himself.'

The whole issue turned into a hopeless confusion just when what the faculty needed was simply to push for its autonomy from the Ministry in a firm and united front. Instead, 'the struggle for Semmelweis' stepped up the conflict that existed before March and split the faculty into two hostile camps. The representatives of these two camps can be gleaned from the signatures on the votes for Klein and Skoda. Skoda's followers, who were in the majority by one vote, were Rokitansky, Dlauthy, Dumreicher, Sigmund, Raimann, and Kainzbauer, and these made up the reform group, while the front against Skoda, and, hence, against the acceptance of Semmelweis's discovery split into two groups: those who believed that the scope of autonomy was being exaggerated, and those who were hostile to reform in general.' They paved the way for a decision from a Ministry in which government conservatism had risen to new heights after the October Revolution that was based on the old regulations.

Rosas' job as provisional vice-director should have been to stand above the fray and provide an objective report to the Ministry. Instead, his introduction to the minutes of the meeting that he gave to the Ministry on February 8, 1849 was an indictment of Skoda that revealed how fatal his actions were. Whether the question was how many associate professors and docents the faculty should have, the title of Skoda's motion, or Semmelweis's discovery, all of which were discussed at the same meeting, this 'yesterday's man' used every question to express his animosity towards 'this new medicine and its most prominent representatives.' The following were the most noteworthy of Rosas' negative references to Semmelweis in the document:

> **[32]** The third feud that appears in Protocol No. III sub 16 and is continued in Protocol IV sub 1, between the professors of medicine and of the first obstetric division, where one of the youngest professors attacks one of the oldest, not in a collegial, friendly manner, but under the guise of scientific research, in truth attacks several colleagues who, having no idea at all of his unfair intention to attack their honor, at first agreed to his proposal. Just as the same endeavor of the same applicant is again shown in N. 2 of Protocol IV, where, with a completely incorrect interpretation of the High Ministerial Decree of 19 December, v. J. Z. 8175 drags down the extraordinary professors and the academic docents, for the purpose of curtailing the rights they first legally acquired from the High Ministry.
>
> The High Ministry wanted to take a lenient view of the pros and cons in order to convince itself of how ineffective one could expect a faculty to be that has among its members those who indulge such ignoble base passions to disturb order and peace at a time when friendly handshakes and vigorous co-operation are necessary to carry out the reforms initiated with the noblest intention by a wise Ministry.
>
> *Vienna 8th February, 1849* *Rosas*
> *suppl. Vicedirector*

'It was certainly not an easy task for the ministerial official responsible for evaluating these materials to arrive at a measured judgment of this complex of questions, suffused as it was with personal resentment and the legal uncertainty of a transitional period. This difficult task fell to Wilhelm von Well (1797-1879), who was of a conservative bent, as F. Allmayerbeck and Hans Lentze's research has shown. Well was vice-director from 1836-1847, director of medical studies from 1847, and became a government advisor and consultant for medical studies in the newly founded Ministry of Education after the revolution. But, despite his conservatism, and to his credit, Well tried and did render the following objective opinion:'

> **[33]** What appears in Protocol No. III sub. 16 and No. IV sub 1 is the continued feud between the professor of medical clinics for physicians and that of the first obstetric division, so it would be very regrettable if desirable scientific research, conducted in the interest of science as well as the health of the woman giving birth, would be abused.
>
> If such research is suggested by a member of the faculty, and recognized by the latter as being timely and useful, the request can only be made to the board of the clinical institute where the same should take place. It would be up to him to take whatever ways and means he considered appropriate for achieving a satisfactory result. He will certainly not refrain from involving those of his colleagues, who can give him help and advice, and conscientiously use every clue that can lead to enlightenment on such an important matter. It is also within the bailiwick of the faculty to be convinced of the accuracy and the reasonableness of the process. It would, however, be as ungracious, as it would exceed the sphere of activity of the faculty, if it wanted to impose on the executive of the first obstetric division, against his will, a commission which was to prescribe investigations and researches at his clinic. This type of procedure would be entirely akin to an inquisition, which may only be initiated by the high authority if there are good reasons to do so.

> However, the Ministry of Public Education finds the scientific research requested by Professor Skoda so important that it wishes itself that it be done in the manner suggested earlier. At the same time it cannot agree with the opinion that at a time when an epidemic does not prevail, nothing can be done to discover the causes of its puzzling appearance, and that a careful and prudent comparison of the more favorable conditions of the present with the unfavorable ones of the past could not elucidate the obscurity in this case……
>
> *Exp. Helft.* *Well*

Schürer von Waldheim failed to construe ('classify') this document correctly because he was not aware either of the February 3 debate by the faculty or the votes cast for Skoda and Klein following the debate, otherwise he would have realized that Well was by no means ready to accept that the faculty had no right to appoint a commission, as argued by the conservative group. On the contrary, Well's report makes it clear that he did recognize such a right only sought in its application to moderate the exaggerated positions of each side.

'Well rejected Skoda's interpretation that the faculty was entitled to appoint a committee and intervene even against the will of the head of a clinic, but also rejected Klein's position that the appointment of a commission in the current, epidemic-free period was pointless. Well, like Skoda, was convinced of the importance of this investigation, but in his opinion it had to be conducted in connection with Klein.'

'Disastrously for Skoda's efforts and Semmelweis's discovery, this part of Well's report was stricken; 'Exp. Helft,' inserted at the end of the stricken portion of Well's report, almost certainly refers to Alexander von Helfert, who was then Undersecretary of Education, and which means that he was responsible for striking this part of Well's report. Helfert's closed-minded view of science and research had its roots in Josephine utilitarianism, and he had made his views clear during the discussions over educational reforms, when Helfert had argued that the School of Surgeons should be retained for the following reasons:

> Medicine, I think, is a science only in its theoretical subjects; in its practical exercise, some illnesses today are a mystery as in

> the days of the Hippocrates. Treatment and healing are empirical and individual geniuses, of which many an old woman, many a son of nature, possessed a richer background than the scholar of the subject.

Thus, the failure of this first attempt to validate Semmelweis's discovery falls squarely on Helfert.'

[35] Semmelweis's Request to Extend his Assistantship

'In previous depictions, Skoda's motion of January 16, 1849 and Semmelweis's request for an extension of the assistantship, which had already been presented to the Vice-director on December 1, 1848, have always been considered separate topics. But if we want to understand the full extent of the struggle for Semmelweis by the group of reformers around Skoda, that is, the representatives of the second Vienna school, then we have to grasp the interrelationship between these two processes on one another, and relate them to other parts of the action. Only such a synoptic view allows one to see that the arguments about both Skoda's motion and the extension of Semmelweis's assistantship were used in the great struggle of a school out of whose soil Semmelweis's discovery grew. Equity requires that this struggle of the Viennese Medical School be given its rightful place in the history of medicine.'

On January 20, 1849, the day that Klein lodged his objection to Skoda's motion, Carl Braun, who was 'a complete novice in obstetrics at the time, submitted an application [at Klein's request, see below] for appointment as Klein's assistant on the first obstetrical division.' On February 17, 1849, Rosas submitted a request to the College of Professors asking 'whether in appointing assistants it was following current norms or the decision of the College on December 9, 1848, by which time Wattman, the then vice-director of education, had already submitted a question about the appointment of assistants to the College in connection with Semmelweis's then pending application, and that the faculty's decision—that the professors in each specialty should have the right to choose assistants, and, therefore, reappointments of assistants also lay with the professors in each specialty— was entirely consistent with the meaning of § 68 of the planned university reform, the draft of which had already been published in July 1848; however, as the matter had still not been decided by the Ministry of Education when Rosas submitted his question to the College, 'it was agreed on February 17th that they should proceed according to the old rules, that is, follow the following procedure: Appraisal of the application by the clinic director (Klein), the vice-director (Rosas), and submission to the study director (Well).' By this ingenious maneuver, Rosas was able to ensure that he and Klein would be completely free to deal with Semmelweis's application independently of the faculty.'

Klein and Rosas submitted reports on February 27 and March 2, respectively, recommending that Carl Braun be appointed Klein's assistant, and that Semmelweis's application be denied. Rosas' recommendation was based on personal consideration, as he argued that the 'lack of harmony between the professor and his assistant make it desirable for the welfare of the institution for Semmelweis to leave.' Klein said nothing about personal conflicts between him and Semmelweis, and instead reproached Semmelweis for having put off other candidates, except Carl Braun, by the confidence he had expressed about his application being granted. 'This was disingenuous and self-serving on Klein's part, because he reproached Semmelweis in order to protect himself from the legitimate rebuke that, he as a hospital director, had not timely provided a successor for his assistant, and, therefore, had to entrust the assistantship at the world's largest obstetric clinic to a complete novice. Up to that time, the assistant's successor had always been appointed provisional assistant up to six months before the assistants changed: Semmelweis became provisional assistant on February 27, 1846, four months before the departure of his predecessor, Breit (July 1, 1846).'

Although Klein and Rosas used different arguments to justify their recommendation, they agreed on one thing: 'that the term of employment of an assistant at the maternity division as on the ophthalmic clinic is limited to one year [sic], so that with his two-year term of office Semmelweis had already exhausted the extension of his assistantship.' This argument was also bogus in as much as 'since 1846 this rule had been honored in the breach on both Klein's division, and on the second division, where Franz Hektor von Arneth's assistantship had been extended to two years. Carl Braun ended up with a four-year assistantship, only—to preserve appearances—his appointment was renewed three times, for one year each time.'

On the very same day (March 2, 1849) that Rosas submitted Semmelweis's request with his and Klein's report to Ministerial Referee, Well acquiesced in the decision to appoint Braun, but distanced himself from the decision with the words: "Should the faculty or, at its waiver of this right, the vice-directorate, suggest in this case that Prof. Klein appoint Braun as assistant to the first obstetric clinic, I shall have no objection to this appointment, provided it has really been already completed." So on 19 March 1849 'Rosas was able to hand his opponent, Skoda, a second defeat.' Not only had Skoda's motion for the appointment of an investigating commission been rejected on February 18th, Semmelweis, for whose sake this commission was to be formed, had to give way. Rosas notified Semmelweis that his application had been denied on March 19, 1849, the last day of his assistantship, with a curt note: "The praiseworthy Medical-Surgical Directorate has not accepted this request. Of which you are hereby informed."

'But the decision on the extension of Semmelweis's assistantship had not yet been taken when, on 23 February 1849, the reform group led by Skoda, representatives of the Second Viennese Medical School, tried one last time to turn things in Semmelweis's favor. They mobilized public opinion from the Forum of the Society of Physicians. The publication organ of this society, the Journal of the Society of Physicians, had already twice been in the service of Semmelweis discovery as Hebra in 1847—for the first time ever—drew attention to it in this organ, and compared its importance to Jenner's cowpox vaccination a few months later. Now, another member, the adjunct director of the General Hospital at that time, Carl Haller (1809-1887), did the same on the basis of the decrease mortality statistics on the first maternity division after Semmelweis introduced chlorine washes. Haller's advocacy for Semmelweis had always been acknowledged as such. It has not yet been recognized that it belonged to the struggle of the Viennese school for Semmelweis. It becomes immediately obvious once we recall Skoda's same undertaking five weeks earlier at the January 16 faculty meeting. But Skoda's statistical proof of the correctness of Semmelweis's doctrine was then presented in the meeting rooms of the faculty and the offices of Well and Helfert, not publicly. When Haller now closed his report before the relevant Viennese medical forum, the Society of Physicians, with the words that the Semmelweis discovery "may certainly be justly recognized by the high state administration," these words were publicly pronounced to that State administration who at the same time had to decide the request of the assistant Semmelweis to extend his service and thus about the further fate of his discovery. Although Haller's report has gone down in the history of medicine as one of the early documents of Semmelweis's discovery, it did not fulfill the function the Vienna School intended in its fight for Semmelweis. The high State administration did not give Semmelweis's discovery the expected recognition. Rather, Semmelweis was dismissed from his assistantship on 19 March by Rosas. Skoda was beaten by his opponent, the vice-director, for a second time. This does not mean, however, that Skoda, the representative par excellence of the absolute in science, abandoned the struggle for Semmelweis and his discovery. Rather, he started it again, and immediately.'

The day after the recommendation to appoint Carl Braun to Semmelweis's post (March 2, 1849), Skoda made a motion at the March 3 meeting of the College whose 'radicalism left nothing to be desired,' namely, that a new vice-director be elected from the professors. Skoda also advised Semmelweis to appeal the denial of his request for an extension of his assistantship. Lesky disagreed with Sinclair that this was bad advice, and rejected as utterly frivolous the analogy that Jakab Bruck had drawn between the fates of Semmelweis and Auenbrugger in Vienna, 'and thus frivolously charged the second Viennese school with collective guilt against Semmelweis. No comparison in the history of medicine would be more inaccurate and unjust than this. van Swieten and De Haen, the leaders of the first Vienna Medical School, hushed up Auenbrugger' new invention; those of the second Viennese school, Hebra, Skoda, Rokitansky Brücke and their students (Arneth, Chiari, Haller, Helm) could not do enough first to announce the discovery of this reticent member of their school, and then to force it onto a world that still fully believed in the genius epidemicus. They wanted to promote him in spite of the anachronistic opposition to every new action. It is all the more praiseworthy considering that nine years later a society as illustrious as the Paris Academy of Medicine, completely rejected Semmelweis's doctrine.

The 'protest' lodged by Theodor Helm (1810-1875), the then provisional director of the General Hospital, 'deserved to be judged as a new action in the battle for Semmelweis. Helm lodged his objection to the appointment of Braun on March 15, 1849, before Semmelweis's assistantship had ended, and his appeal had been filed. Helm had begun his career as an obstetrician and had himself written a well-publicized monograph on puerperal fever (1839). He handed his objection to the medical faculty, not the vice-director, and to the Lower Austrian Provincial Government. His objection to Braun's appointment was based on the fact that it had violated the established principle of first appointing a provisional assistant on the first maternity clinic, and therefore, Braun's appointment could not ensure the proper care of women giving birth at this clinic because Braun had not received sufficient training in obstetrics:'

[42] From the Imperial Hospital Administration
Note

It is doubtless known to the most worthy faculty, how much whatever happens in the area of the hospital, be it really remarkable or at least accepted as such, reflects on the institution itself and its public honor. This applies no less to the clinics than to the ordinary wards, in that the greater public is not aware of their separate and necessary supervision and direction, and, therefore, it is easier to consider any clinical procedure as from the hospital and its leadership, without the same or its leadership being more involved in it.

It is just as well known to the commendable leading faculty that until now the assistants on the maternity division' had been appointed several months before their actual service. In the meanwhile, they should be able to acquire the necessary practical knowledge in order to be able to provide the most urgent, even immediate, practical assistance in many cases.

It has therefore disconcerted the undersigned Director that the appointment of the former internist of the General Hospital,

> Dr. Braun, was a departure from this practice in that he is to begin his functions on the 19th of this month.
>
> The Director, therefore, wanted to draw the attention of the worthy faculty to this fact, to insure itself against all eventualities...[26] has the honour to report it notified the high state government, as its highest authority, of this note.
>
> *Vienna, 15 March, 1849.* *Helm.*
>
> To the worthy senior faculty of medical and surgical studies, on the Imperial University of Vienna.

Klein rejected Helm's complaint in the harshest terms in a response dated March 27, 1849, but the text of Klein's response was not reproduced in the monograph 'because his arguments were repeated in Klein's March 28, 1849 response to Semmelweis's petition appealing the denial of his application and dismissal as assistant.' Semmelweis's petition has been lost but 'the main points of its content could be reconstructed from Bartsch's report, and with respect to Semmelweis's petitions, as Well was no longer dealing only with Klein's opinions as Franz Bartsch (1800-1861), Klein's colleague who headed the second maternity division also became involved in the matter. Bartsch was one of Klein's former assistants, and had signed Klein's January 20 objection to Skoda's motion. The following is text of his report concerning Semmelweis's application for an extension of his assistantship:'

> **[43]** Statement of the undersigned concerning the report from the high Ministry of Education to the medical faculty on the request of the assistant to the first maternity clinic, Dr. Semmelweis, to extend his appointment for a further two years.
>
> Dr. Semmelweis supports his request with the following reasons:
>
> 1. He believes he has discovered the cause of childbed fever and, through the experiments he employed, to have significantly reduced the high mortality rates that had taken place on the first

[26] The ellipsis indicates damage to the text.

maternity clinic in earlier years, and therefore wishes to continue his research in this area in the interests of science.

2. His successor to be, Dr. Braun, was appointed only 14 days ago, instead of 6 months before as usual until now, is thus unable to take on the position of assistant at such a large institution, where often instantaneous assistance is required.

As to the first, as far as the undersigned knows, Dr. Semmelweis came to the conclusion that childbed fever was caused by a contagious substance transferred by the practitioners from the autopsy room to the birth house, wherefore on the recommendation made to the professor, the practitioners were instructed by the latter, to wash their hands before they go to women in labor with chlorine water instead of soap as before. Although during the time these chlorine washings were taking place on the first delivery clinic, namely, in 1848, the mortality there was very low, the great value attributed to them may still be doubted because (a) at the same time a much more favorable Genius epidemicus was so prevalent among women that in the course of 4 months no significant sickenings and not a single death occurred on the second obstetric clinic; because (b) the said chlorine washings were only introduced after the epidemic ceased, and (c) because on the division for midwives, who don’t come into contact with the death chamber at all, the most vicious forms of puerperal fever still occurred at certain times. Nevertheless, the undersigned believes that these chlorine washes should be continued to investigate their supposed effects, which will more certainly happen, as before, under the direction of the professor that ordered it without yielding as yet definite results, and for whom the welfare of the institution is closest to his heart. It is therefore not clear that an extension of the period of Dr. Semmelweis’s service is necessary for this purpose.

As to the second, the previous custom of appointing assistants to this institution 6 months before their service actually began, stemmed from the time when the assistants often did not obtain their Master of Obstetrics before their service, and, moreover, there was only one maternity division, and the professor had to live outside the hospital. But now the circumstances have changed so much that the Assistant must already have their Master of Obstetrics by the time of their appointment, and so must be able to practice as such; furthermore, there are currently two divisions, and these have the obligation to support each other in the event of illness of the professor as well as in urgent matters of service; finally the professor lives in the institution itself, and so does more in case of an emergency than Dr. Semmelweis portrays.

Although an extension of Dr. Semmelweis's service is by no means necessary for the reasons stated in the petition, the same could nevertheless be granted if the professor was satisfied with his previous service and conduct, which, however, does not seem to be the case, because the professor did not recommend this extension of service.

Incidentally, the undersigned believes that one must stick to the resolution passed unanimously by the medical faculty, according to which the choice of assistants, as well as the possible extensions of their service, is entirely up to the professors, since they alone are responsible for the institutes entrusted to them.

Vienna, March 25, 1849 *Prof. Bartsch*

Bartsch and Klein's reports provided 'a good insight' into the grounds on which Semmelweis's proof of his theory was rejected by 'the Viennese anti-Semmelweis front:' they argued that the epidemic had already ceased by the time the 'chlorwashings' were first introduced and, therefore, Semmelweis had by no means definitively established its value because he had not proved that 'the prevailing favorable genius epidemicus [was not] to be thanked for the much lower mortality rate.' Bartsch was the 'spiritual father' of the idea that may have hurt the spread of the Semmelweis discovery even more than its harsh rejection: namely, 'the idea of retaining the practical consequences of the discovery, i.e. the chlorine-washing, while at the same time attacking the theoretical premises of Semmelweis's doctrine.' Bartsch's former assistant, Eduard

Lumpe (1813-1876), who became a docent in Obstetrics in Vienna, and Semmelweis opponent, later characterized this policy as 'Wait and Wash.'

'Klein's March 28, 1849 report on Semmelweis's appeal of the denial of his application, was as follows:'

[45] Pro Memoria

After hearing that Dr. Semmelweis took action on receiving notification of the negative decision of the Vice-director of the high ministry of Education on the extension of his assistantship, the undersigned allows himself to obediently submit to the Undersecretary his ideas against such an extension:

a. The Professor of the 1st Obstetrical Division directs his institution, as do the other clinical professors their institutions, the assistant is his assistant, the institution is handed over to the professor, only he is responsible for it, so it cannot be handed over to his assistant either directly or indirectly, because he himself is not responsible.

b. For the chlorine washings on the 1st Obstetrical Divisions, which the Professor ordered and introduced at the suggestion of his assistant, to continue in order to learn if these prevented the recurrence of an epidemic, the professor of this division took care that the determination of the cause and prevention of the epidemic must first and foremost lie at its heart.

c. The pretense that the institution must suffer because qualifications of the newly appointed assistant for this service are inadequate, is therefore unfounded, because the professor, not the assistant, directs the institute, who lives in the institution, and can be summoned just as quickly as the assistant to aid in the case of an immediate emergency. Also, in case the professor becomes ill, and other absences are taken care of by the professors of the two obstetric clinics who cover for each other.

d. The custom of naming an assistant six months before the commencement of his service so they can be better qualified was written at a time when there was only one obstetric division, and only one professor of the same, who besides lived outside the institution and thus could neither be summoned so quickly nor be supplemented by a second professor in the same field; and in the event of the death or unexpected departure of the assistant, the professor had to manage all this with a newly appointed one. By the way, this time the Assistant could not be appointed earlier because Dr. Semmelweis's statement that his assistantship would be extended without doubt deterred all previous ones, and Dr. Braun only competed in the last minute.

e. It is by no means clear from the fact that since the termination of the last epidemic of childbed fever the mortality rate is lower, that it is the result of chlorine washes, that the cause of the childbed epidemic has been found, and its recurrence was prevented. For this the experiment is still too young, and therefore the appropriation of so much merit by Semmelweis is still premature and presumptuous.

f. Finally, Dr. Semmelweis' behavior, so presumptuous and arbitrary in reliance on this supposed merit, and the zealous support of his friends in the faculty, contradicted his instructions: he operated on his own initiative; he operated on nothing less than urgent cases, delayed cases shortly before ward rounds just to give the professor the opportunity to operate and demonstrate to his students. He forbade nurses and midwives to report to the professor during his ward rounds on concealed parts of the body, he did not obey instructions and ordered the opposite. So a child died at the beginning of March of adhesion of the anus, which condition could not be detected because the enemas ordered by the professor and others also for the purpose of discovering organic defects of the anus were not followed, indeed, even forbidden.

Such conduct by Dr. Semmelweis, the Assistant, completely ignored the work of the Professor for the good of the institution in general, and was contrary to public education in particular, and also the interest of humanity, the latter could not be expected to agree to extend the Assistenship of the former, because he would obviously violate the duties expected of him. The undersigned also hopes that the high ministry will not want to embitter his years of service with an Assistant hostile to him, with whom it would be impossible for him to serve without sacrificing his health.

Vienna, March 28, 1849. *Dr. J. Klein*
Prof. of 1. Birthclinic

The literature has so far only outlined the facts of Klein's report, but in the present context, one of its many facets needed to be highlighted: namely, the discrepancy between the reasons Klein gave in this report for denying Semmelweis's application and those he had given in his report of February 27, 1849, and especially the fact that in his earlier report, Klein had not criticized Semmelweis's performance as assistant, whereas in his subsequent report (of March 28), Klein went to great lengths to lay out all the shortcomings and deficiencies of Semmelweis's performance as assistant, as this explained what Rosas had meant by the 'lack of harmony' between the professor and his assistant in his March 2, report. Klein must have had some good reason for deeming it advisable to avoid passing judgment on Semmelweis's performance as assistant in his report of 27 February, and for criticizing Semmelweis's performance, and compiling everything he could to bring against his assistant only after Semmelweis's had appealed to the Ministry. 'But what kind of inhibitions were these?'

'Fortunately, we have a document—one that has so far escaped discovery by earlier research on Semmelweis—that not only clarifies this question, but allows us to understand the forces deployed in the struggle against Semmelweis. Klein must have felt the need to explain the discrepancies between his two reports, as he submitted this document as a supplement to his March 28, 1849 report to the Ministry on the same day as his report:'

[48] Supplement C

Finally, the undersigned must also note that on November 19 of last year, he gave Dr. Semmelweis, who in the course of the previous year had repeatedly acted contrary to his instructions and had already earned the dissatisfaction of his professor, a favorable report on his service at his request. But Dr. Semmelweis rewarded the undersigned badly for this message, and from the time he received the testimony, he thought he now had in his hands the means to cover himself against the complaints of the undersigned, disregard his duties, and disobeyed the instructions given to him; the undersigned very much regrets his leniency towards Dr. Semmelweis, and to have given him such a favorable testimony, which, truthfully, he could no longer do.

'We find out from this supplement an important and most surprising detail: namely, that on November 19, 1848, Klein had given Semmelweis a very good, even "so favorable" a reference that he was now forced to reconcile the contradiction between that reference and the serious accusations Klein levelled against Semmelweis in his 28 March 1849 report.' One can assume that Semmelweis attached Klein's favorable reference to his December 1, 1848 application, and that on November 19, 1848, when Wattman was still the vice-director of medical education, Klein was still willing to keep his assistant who he had described so favorably on at his clinic for a further two years. This is consistent with the certainty with which Semmelweis spoke to others about the extension of his assistantship that Klein referred to several times.

'There is, therefore, no doubt that between November 19, 1848 and January 20, 1849, the day on which Klein protested against Skoda's motion, and asked Carl Braun to submit an application, Klein made a disastrous about-turn and abandoned his plan to extend Semmelweis's assistantship. On December 30, the Vice-director changed. On the same day, Rosas took over the leadership of the matter, and in January immediately started his fight against the reformer, Skoda, on a broad front, as the minutes of the various meetings show. Klein first became Semmelweis's opponent in this fight' and was not ill-disposed towards Semmelweis before that as less critical historical research has portrayed him to be. Semmelweis's request was drawn into this fights in which Rosas exercised the full extent of the vice-directorial power.'

'That is how at the meeting of the medical faculty on March 31, 1849 there were, in addition to Semmelweis's appeal, two reports written by Klein and Bartsch. Semmelweis's complaint was heard first, and then the protagonists faced off. The conservative group under the Rosas's leadership insisted on the right of every professor to extend the service of his assistant, whereas the reformers tried once again to form a commission. This time it was Rokitansky, the giant of Viennese medicine; the time was 1849, thirty years before Rokitansky's Berlin colleague, Rudolf Virchow, would recognize the significance of Semmelweis's discovery. The minutes of the March 31, 1849 meeting indicated that Rokitansky used the dispute over Semmelweis's request for an extension of his assistantship as an argument for appointing a commisssion:'

> '... Doctor Semmelweis has shown such merit that he deserves the extension. But as the disagreements between him and his professor are such as to call into question these achievements, which are highly important to science and humanity, it calls for the composition of a commission, which has the task to explore the situation both in the interest of Professor Klein and the Dr. Semmelweis as well as science.'

'Helm's protest against Braun's appointment next came up for discussion, and this time it was again Skoda who opposed Rosas by insisting that the tried and tested practice of having assistants on the maternity clinic first work there provisionally should not be dispensed with without first consulting the faculty on the matter. But the Ministry and its Undersecretary, Joseph Alexander Helfert, had the last word. On April 9, 1849, they handed down the decision on Semmelweis's assistantship, and repeated it again on May 13, after Helm's objection to Braun's appointment had already been rejected on April 16. Thus, all parts of the sweeping offensive for the implementation of Semmelweis's teaching that the Viennese school had started in January 1849, collapsed in April. The individual actors, above all Skoda, had suffered heavy defeats. Semmelweis himself was deprived of effectiveness in his field (*Wirkungsfeldes beraubt*). But this campaign did achieve one thing: the Ministry had become uncertain through the numerous expert reports, and the negative attitudes in the opposing expert opinions. This is evidenced by a Ministerial Decree of 8 April 1849 that used the minutes of that furious meeting on 10 February in a remarkable way. Helfert emphasized the remarks concerning the decree of 18 February about the dispute over the establishment of a commission requested by Skoda, but then, quite unexpectedly, adds the directive: "incidentally, the two professors of obstetrics, Klein and Bartsch, strongly urge, and hold the clinical assistants and chief midwives responsible that the chlorine washings are applied punctually and conscientiously, since part of the faculty considers them effective preventative against infection of women in labor from touching." Many obstetricians later made 'waiting and washing' their motto. It had been officially decreed at the obstetric clinics of Vienna since 8 April 1849.'

'In this fight, we have seen the various members of the Viennese school one after another advocate for Semmelweis, especially Skoda. With his small, stocky build, soft voice, there was certainly nothing heroic about him, and yet he was the hero of this fight. Haller, Helm, and Rokitansky had spoken for Semmelweis, made objections and motions, and Dumreicher, Dlauthy, Sigmuch, Raimann, and Kainzbauer gave their voice. Only one did not show up in the bitter struggle for the greatest discovery of the Vienna School: Semmelweis himself. On February 23, in a time of great tension, the Society of Physicians invited him to speak about his discovery. But Semmelweis has remained silent. He did not comment on his discovery either orally or in writing, and thereby made his already difficult fight even harder for his friends. It was as Sinclair has already noted: "besides Rosas and Klein, Semmelweis was his own worst enemy."'

[52] Lectures for Oral Examinations

'It is an apt reflection of the confused state of the Semmelweis literature over the connections illuminated here that no one until now has even asked, let alone tried to answer, how Semmelweis occupied himself in Vienna from the time of his dismissal from the first maternity division clinic on March 19, 1849 until his departure to Budapest in mid-October, 1850, which is, after all, 1½ years. It is impossible for the nine animal experiments that Skoda referred to in his lecture to the Academy to have filled his time. We must thank Rosas for an act of vice-directorial arbitrariness on April 26, 1849 in the files for shedding at least a partial light on this question.'

The backdrop to these events was the dissolution of the Joseph Military Medical Academy in 1848, following which, the Ministry of Education had committed to the Ministry of Defense on November 25, 1848 that those pupils who had not completed their studies could finish them at the university. These 'Josphiners,' as they were referred to, applied to the chief medical officer for reimbursement of 50 Gulden for the various courses they had taken for their oral examinations. Since the chief medical office had been assured that these students would be provided education free, he understandably asked for clarification from the vice-directorate. Rosas, without making any inquiries to the faculty, expressed his astonishment that these pupils were 'taking lessons from individuals to whom they were not assigned, and who they had to pay,' while equally competent, if not more capable, men would have given such lessons for free.

After his assistantship ended, Semmelweis earned part of his keep by giving courses for oral examinations to the Josephiners, which may occasionally have been followed by practical obstetrics, presumably on cadavers made available to Semmelweis by Rokitansky. Rosas commented that 'obstetrical (courses) at the maternity clinic are more profitably given by assistant Dr. Braun than Semmelweis (and not for 10 florins). 'The postscript "that the complaining academic pupils either did not know the conditions, or, what is more probable, were tempted to their costly decisions by money-hungry people and their accomplices," leaves not the slightest doubt about the nature of Rosas's sentiments towards Semmelweis.' The 'remarkable aftermath' of this tawdry affair further illustrated the 'fighting spirit of the Second Vienna Medical School.'

On May 12, 1849, Skoda, Rokitansky, Dumrecicher, Raimann, Kainzbauer, and this time also Shuh, protested this new affront to the autonomy of the faculty directly to the Ministry. 'After all, Rosas had dared to go above heads of the College of Professors to a non-departmental authority (*bereichsfremden Behörde*), such as chief medical officer of the Ministry of Defense, to attack the reputation and honor of former students, now so-called emeritus assistants, Semmelweis and Blodig, by using the title "emeritus" in such a scornful way. The same professors decided collectively to ask the Ministry of Education that if such an office was to continue to exist, its occupant should no longer have a seat or voice within the faculty. We reproduce at least the second part of the text of this impressive document:'

> **[53]** Given the comments of the provisional vice-director that the supplicants were tempted by the malicious impulses of money-hungry people and their accomplices, to attend the courses of these gentlemen, the undersigned must lodge a protest; these comments contain the slander of men who enjoy a perfectly honorable reputation; this remark prostitutes the school where we work; this remark is incomprehensible, because the assistants are not bound by the existing regulations to give free courses—the two, Semmelweis and Blodig, are emeritus assistants. Only the good reputation, which the courses of these men have rightly earned, motivated the supplicants to attend the courses of these men. The petitioners were also not prevented by the lack of money to get lessons for their rigorous examinations in these courses, because the gentlemen mentioned have given petitioners access to their courses for a month, and are not at all accustomed to demand a fee from their listeners. There was therefore no grounds, on the part of the provisional vice-director, to issue an order without the consent of the faculty, that, in addition to lacking expert knowledge, contains obvious falsehoods, bears the stamp of spite, and would not be wrongly called abuse of official power ...
>
> The undersigned believe that a High Ministry cannot approve of this kind of management of the office of the provisional vice-director, and if such management of the office were allowed in the future, they would ask a high ministry to dispense with the seat and say of the same within the faculty.
>
> *Vienna on 12 May, 1849*
>
> *Prof. Schuh*
> *Prof. Skoda*
> *Prof. Suppl. Dumreicher*
> *Prof. Raimann*
> *Prof. Suppl. Dr. Kainzbauer*
> *Prof. Rokitansky*

'Undersecretary Helfert replied to this protest on July 9, 1849 when the semester was already coming to an end. The most disastrous vice-directorate that ever existed while the office was in existence was also coming to an end. And it is not to Helfert's credit that he condoned Rosas's arbitrariness, and held that in all respects he, Rosas, and not the professors, was in the right: "Abuse of official power or the slander of individuals or even of the entire faculty cannot be blamed on the vice-director," are the words with which on 9 July 1849, Helfert sealed the third defeat of the Viennese school in the battle for Semmelweis.'

[55] The Methodical Requirements of Semmelweis's Discovery

'It testifies to the relentless fighting spirit and at the same time to the profound sense of responsibility that Skoda and the men around him had for Semmelweis's discovery that, despite all their defeats, they resumed the fight immediately when a change in the political situation became apparent. Although Helfert remained Undersecretary of Education, Count Leo Thun - Hohenstein (1811-1888), whose name is associated with the great educational reform in Austria, took over the leadership of the Ministry of Education. On September 30, 1849, the provisional law on the organization of the academic authorities was enacted. With this law, the office of deputy director ceased to exist. The self-administration was now transferred in a clearly identifiable way to the College of Professors. On October 1, 1849, Carl Rokitansky, Semmelweis's teacher, became the first freely elected dean of the medical school. A new, large-scale offensive for Semmelweis had already began on 18 October 1849 with the penetrating reflection of Skoda's lecturer, which he held that day before the country's highest scientific forum country, the Imperial Academy of Sciences, "On Dr. Semmelweis's discovery of the true nature of the unusually high occurrence of a common disease of women in the Viennese birth house, and the means of reducing this disease down to its usual number."'

'Again and again, since January 16, 1849, we have encountered Skoda as the main campaigner for Semmelweis. So it may now be time to ask why he adopted Semmelweis's cause in such a personal way. Certainly, his struggle for Semmelweis was inextricably linked to the realization of university autonomy with which Skoda was concerned, as previously described. But beyond that, Skoda adopted Semmelweis's discovery in a way as if it was his own business. This personal commitment can only be understood from the special relationship in which Skoda **[56]** stood to Semmelweis as Semmelweis's devotee—Klein called him Skoda's partisan [*Parteigänger*]. However, Semmelweis was more than Skoda's devotee. He was his pupil in the very pristine sense of the word.'

'If we take the full extent of this student-teacher relationship seriously, and take from it the full methodological consequences for Semmelweis's discovery, we will complete the essential outlines of the conventional image of Semmelweis. For in this picture, all light is gathered on the ingenious discoverer, who is presented as a unique phenomenon standing apart from his time. However, we want to bring Semmelweis back into the milieu of his school and the ground from which his discovery grew, and confront the often-discussed question of what Vienna owes Semmelweis and compared with what he owed to Vienna's medical school. The answer can only be: from a scientific point of view, all the methodological means that were a prerequisite for his discovery.'

'Once we consider this discovery in terms of its methodological constituents, we can highlight three prongs: 1. The pathological-anatomical precondition; 2. A very specific final comparative-analytic procedure, which Sinclair characterized well as 'Elimination of Factors,' and 3. crowning it all, the statistical proof.'

'As for the pathological-anatomical premise of Semmelweis's discovery, this was placed in the correct light by E. F. Podach, and his advanced work on the structure of puerperal-anatomy. Although he has deprived Semmelweis's discovery of its romantic aura of a lightening, accidental discovery in connection with the Kolletschka case, he made visible for the first time the hard pathologic-anatomical work that Semmelweis had actually done. Podach showed that it required years of training and experience in systematic pathologic-anatomical thinking until Semmelweis was able to override the view of his teacher Rokitansky of the supposed puerperal **[57]** specificity of pyaemia, and to view the anatomical changes in the corpses of mothers and their newborns, as well as those in Kolletschka's corpse, as one pyemia. If Semmelweis essentially arrived at his new version of the term "puerperal fever" in this synopsis of the pathological-anatomy, and in this went beyond Rokintansky, he was still only able to do this through the training in systematic pathological-anatomical thinking he received from him.'

'But Semmelweis was also able to combine what he recognized morphologically into an etiological and clinical entity. In this tripartite correlation, the correctness of the Rokitansky-Skoda school received its broadest support in Semmelweis's discovery. Otherwise it was only given to this school to connect anatomically established facts with findings in the living, and to evaluate them diagnostically. Skoda developed a special final method for this that the lecturer from Tübingen, Carl Wunderlich, had described six years before Semmelweis's discovery (1841) as follows: "Dismissing inessential, irrelevant phenomena that had so often been referred as pathognomonic in the past, and crediting clinical findings only in so far as they were demonstrably related in a comprehensible way, physical, or physiological, to material change." Wunderlich had pointed out that one and the same phenomenon could have fundamentally different causes and that "the task with every diagnostic question is to take into account all possibilities, and only decide on an interpretation by exclusion or by predominant probability."'

'Skoda developed this "exclusion procedure" or the "diagnosis per exclusionem," the name by which it has entered the history of medicine, **[58]** into a teachable and learnable method, and passed it on to his students in such a precise way that Viennese internists in the second half of the 19th century became famous throughout Europe for their "lightening-diagnosis" based on this procedure.'

'But Semmelweis was not only one of the most eager visitors to Skoda's lectures; in order to be fully aware of what he meant for Semmelweis's methodical training, it also needs to be carefully considered, that from October 10, 1844, until he became Klein's provisional assistant to on February 27, 1846, i.e. for almost one and a half years, he attended as praeparandus externus VI. Medical Department and the associated division for chest diseases continuously to the greatest satisfaction of his master, Primarius Skoda. And when Skoda was appointed professor in October 1846, Semmelweis would have most liked to join him as Assistant, so great and so strong was the influence that teacher exerted on him. As an intimate pupil, Semmelweis had almost a year and a half opportunity to get to know the method of exclusion technique, the core of his diagnostic training, directly from the master himself, and to practice it daily under his control.'

'Semmelweis transferred this sophisticated comparative exclusion technique that Skoda developed in the field of diagnosis to the etiology field, and with its help solved the problem that struck him in the spring of 1847, the high mortality of women delivering on the first maternity division, which his sensitive soul made the problem his own: why did three times as many women die on this, the medical division, than on the second maternity division, the midwives' division?'

'This eerie difference had troubled the heads of governmental commissions, and raised hypotheses upon hypotheses: weather influences, **[59]** the genius epidemicus in particular; overcrowding and bad ventilation of the rooms, their year-long infection with "puerperal miasma;" the anxiety of the newly delivered on the deadly first maternity division; clinic; yes, even the wounded feeling of shame of women at being examined by students, and, above all, the medical treatment on this division were all to blame for this gruesome difference in mortality. Skoda's student, Semmelweis, thinned this jungle of fictitious etiologies by exercising the method of exclusion he learned from his master. He distinguished one possibility listed above after the other, and in a comparative analysis he checked specifically whether the factors cited were able to account for the difference in mortality in a satisfactory, that is to say scientifically based way. Finally, there was only one option left: infection of the birth parts (*Geburtsteile*) by cadaveric-poison on the unwashed fingers of doctors and students.'

'Until now, the main credit for the discovery of childbed fever had been too lightly given to the bad gymnasium in Ofen, the bad school that had allowed Semmelweis's ingenious gift to develop freely, so that "his bright mind could explain the observed with playfulness in the simplest possible way, while learned minds could not see what his eye revealed ..." That the sophisticated, multi-faceted thought process Semmelweis learned in his daily dealings with the master of diagnostic reasoning, and applied in a creative way to his problem, could only be the product of a mind unprepared in school to a historical account unconcerned with medical historiography. Thus has the way been blocked to a real appreciation of Semmelweis's achievement in uncovering the true cause of child bed fever, an achievement that in truth presents itself as an ingenious integration of different methods of thinking and working. For the premises of this discovery are not yet exhausted with the previously outlined pathological-anatomical conditions and application of the exclusion method. Semmelweis learned in Skoda's rigorous school that a diagnosis can only claim credibility if it has been proven pathologico- **[60]** anatomically. So his results, obtained by means of the comparative-analytic exclusion procedure, namely, that the fingers of the doctors and students that were contaminated with cadaveric poison caused the puerperal epidemic at the first maternity division, had to be proven. Here, too, it was taken for granted that Semmelweis's statistical proof was based on the extensive mortality and morbidity tables, without anyone ever asking how the use of the numerical-statistical method came to him.'

'In the application of this method too, Semmelweis proved himself to be a faithful student of Skoda. Just as Skoda strove for a precise scientific foundation of his diagnoses, he also sought the same for his therapeutic actions. He found them among the Parisian clinicians, Louis and Andral, who, in order to determine whether a drug had value or was worthlessness, employed comparative serial experiments in patients in their clinics and analyzed them statistically.'

'Just at the time when Semmelweis was Skoda's "praeperandus externus," the latter was particularly concerned with trying to obtain statistical substantiation for his therapy. Let us hear what a contemporary doctor reported about it in 1847: "As concerns the treatment Skoda was practicing in his department, and which he is perhaps now using at the clinic, I want first to mention that Skoda, as far as I know, followed a numerical method, and, therefore, he gave certain remedies for certain diseases for a long time, then abandoned it, then for a long time used another remedy, then another, and so on, and, finally, compared the results in those who died and recovered."'

'So there can be no doubt that Semmelweis, in addition to the exclusion method, also learned to handle the statistical method from

Skoda, and transplanted it from the therapeutic to the aetiological area. But while Skoda, in the undeveloped form in which he practiced statistics in the therapeutic field, did not have much luck with it, it **[61]** proved itself to be the solution to etiological problem of his pupil, Semmelweis. All he had to do was compare the mortality statistics of both maternity divisions, and the numbers made the correctness of his hypothesis immediately evident, at least to any unprejudiced person, namely: that there was a much greater possibility of transferring decaying animal-organic matter on the doctors division than on the midwives' division.'

'So we have got to know Semmelweis as a student of Skoda in a methodologically very concrete way. By combining his methods with Rokitansky's pathological-anatomical reasoning, and employing them ingeniously to solve his special question about the cause of the difference in mortality between the two divisions, he attained a new synthesis: the discovery of the true cause of childbed fever. Skoda, with the inner evidence of spiritual co-authorship, immediately recognized in this new, genuine product of those methods of investigation and thought that Rokitansky and he had so distinctly imprinted on their school. Therefore, as we know from the written justification of his petition of January 20, 1849 (sic) and from his Academy lecture, that he felt, to the highest degree, responsible to science and humanity, to ensure that this intellectual property of the Viennese school took its place in science and obstetrical practice. And all the more so since the discoverer himself, Semmelweis, despite the invitation of the Society of Physicians on February 23, remained silent. So Skoda felt it his task after the failure of the first offensive on behalf of Semmelweis's theory to open a new one for him. He did this with his lecture to the Academy 18 October 18, 1849. This lecture has always been taken to be, what it also is, as the first detailed presentation of Semmelweis's discovery. Let us now grasp that it was more than just a presentation, also more than the prelude to a new offensive: as Skoda traced, step by step, the path to Semmelweis's discovery (*Erkenntnisweg*) in front of the Academy, he at the same time demonstrated with his presentation a classic example of the ingenious application of his own method of working and thinking.'

[62] Application for Docentur

'We have previously highlighted the School's share in the inner methodology of Semmelweis' discovery, especially in connection with Skoda's Academy-lecture. Now we want to ask: what was the tactical purpose of this lecture in the battle for Semmelweis? To anticipate: the same purpose as Haller's lecture to the Society of Physicians on February 23rd: to demonstrate to the world the importance of Semmelweis's discovery, and especially to emphasize by the demonstration where it took place.'

'If the country's highest scientific forum happily took up and showed its interest in Semmelweis's discovery—as it did by the actual grant of a sum of money for animal experiments—one might have expected this attitude to have had an effect on the conservative civil servants and Semmelweis-opponents by serving as an example. After all, other men had risen to head the authorities: Thun in the Ministry of Education and Rokitansky in the medical College of Professors; but here and there, there were still enough representatives of the conservative mind-set. Helfert and Well were, successively, undersecretaries in the Ministry. Rosas, who spoke on behalf of medical education in the College, although deprived of his vice-directorship, was still the intellectual centre of the Viennese anti-Semmelweis front. We have earlier already touched on their inhomogeneous structure. In addition to Semmelweis's dogmatic opponents, there were those who did not feel committed to the situation, and when the situation changed, as with the law created on September 30, 1849, they wanted to disengage themselves, once it was made emphatically clear to them that the Viennese Academy of Sciences stood behind Semmelweis's discovery.'

[63] It is not a coincidence, but only confirms the opinion expressed here about the tactical function of Skoda's Academy lecture, that Semmelweis waited for it to appear in print before he submitted his *habilitation.* This was on February 9, 1850: that day Semmelweis submitted his request for *habilitation* to the College of Professors, which had the following wording:

Praiseworthy Medical Faculty of the College of Professors!

The respectful undersigned asks the praiseworthy College to examine his qualifications for a Docentur of theoretical obstetrics for surgeons and physicians with demonstration of phantoms and cadavers, and in the event that the praiseworthy College should decide in favor of the worthiness of the most devoted petitioner, to expedite the submission to the high Ministry of Education. This request is supported by the following rationale:

1. The undersigned is, according to supplements A, B, C, Doctor of Medicine and Surgery, and Master of Obstetrics.

2. Since 1844, the same has occupied himself with the study and practice of obstetrics, and during this time was, for 2 years, an Assistant on the first maternity clinic. D. E. F. The quality of the services required by this position hardly needs discussion before this praiseworthy College, and their quality with respect to the most devoted petitioner is confirmed by the satisfactory testimonies of Professor Klein. D. E. F.

3. The obedient undersigned, during the time of his service as Assistant, gave private lessons and lectures on theoretical and practical obstetrics to more than 300 students, and thereby has already proved the skills required for public lectures.

4. The undersigned believes that in the enclosed manuscript G. he has given evidence that in the field of obstetrics, he is capable of handling both the theoretical and practical parts of his science in a manner appropriate to the times.

5. The research of the obedient undersigned on the genesis and nature of so-called puerperal fever—which has already been appreciated by the Imperial Academy of Sciences, H. 1-2—might on this occasion also be recognized by the praiseworthy College of Professors, and **[64]** considered worthy to be recommended to the high Ministry.

6. The undersigned encloses a curriculum vitae, J, and a program, K, on the nature of the lectures to be delivered, and, therefore,

believes that everyone will be allowed to start normal lectures in the Summer semester.

Vienna February 9, 1850 *Dr. Ignaz Semmelweis*

The remarkable fact about this application was that Semmelweis did not use his discovery for his *habilitation* thesis—even though 'there could truly have been no better doctoral thesis than that on the etiology, the concept, and the prophylaxis of childbed fever.' Instead, 'the incomprehensible waverer' submitted fragmentary essays on some modifications of surgical obstetrical techniques the novelty of which might or might not be accepted, and first referred to his research "on the genesis and nature of so-called puerperal fever" as the penultimate, fifth item. The full significance of Skoda's lecture to the Academy could be appreciated from the fact that Semmelweis attached the lecture, together with the letter from the Academy awarding Semmelweis a grant to conduct animal experiments, as supplements H. 1-2 to his application.

'One can see the effect of Skoda's careful action from the February 15, 1850 report of Franz Bartsch, professor on the [second] midwives's division.' In his comments on Semmelweis's request for an extension of his assistantship a year earlier, Bartsch had only negative things to say about Semmelweis's discovery, but now **[65]** 'he dared not attack Semmelweis's habilitation application with even a single word.' Bartsch not only approved Semmelweis's *habilitation* without more, but with regard to its scientific and practical assessment, even advocated waiving the *habilitation viva voce*, being satisfied with him just giving a trial lecture, from which 'an incipient softening of the anti-Semmelweis front was apparent.'

When Semmelweis gave this trial lecture on February 23, 1850, it became apparent that 'the old front against Semmelweis would try to stir.' The week before, Klein had asked Rokintansky for Semmelweis's application and Bartsch's report, and he now expressed reservations about Semmelweis's *habilitation* thesis both orally and in writing, saying that it was not suitable as a supplement, which Rokitansky recorded in his minutes of the meeting with: "One part of the college (sees) the matter as a private one, and the other larger part regards it as an improper transaction." Nevertheless, at the same session, it was decided to hold a colloquium with Semmelweis the next day, February 24th, and, surprisingly, Semmelweis's followers approved this, despite their original decision to waive the colloquium. They did this in order to give Semmelweis an opportunity to respond to Klein's reservations about his *habilitation* thesis, as on February 17, 1850, the Ministry had already issued a decree to the Dean's office, in connection with the rejection of the *habilitation* application of another candidate, the Viennese syphilisologist Hermann Zeissl (1817-1884), that prescribed an extremely strict *habilitation* for the College. After Semmnelweis's colloquium, Bartsch, obviously under Klein's influence, softened his positive report of 15 February, and stated in a separate report on February 24th that Semmelweis was fully qualified for the Docentur, but added that 'Dr. Semmelweis's specified modification (*Wendung auf den Kopf*) cannot be recognized as a **[66]** new operation as it had not only been practiced for many years at the local maternity hospital, but also described as cumbersome by Dr. Lumpe in his work, "A Course on Obstetrics."' However, the majority of the College accepted Semmelweis's modification as new.

'On March 2, Rokitansky submitted to the Ministry the College's proposal to "confer a Docentur on Dr. Semmelweis for theoretical obstetrics with demonstrations on phantoms and cadavers." Rokitansky added a comment to his introduction that shows that he foresaw the coming difficulties even then, and attempted to deal with it at the outset by stating in his submission to the Ministry, as regards the presently available teaching materials, which petitioners have referred to as phantoms, it would be easier instead to give the cadavers from the autopsy room of the hospital to the docents rather than to use them elsewhere. This laid out the so-called "cadaver question," which had such a decisive role in the denouement of Semmelweis's docentur.'

Lesky then digressed to clear up the confusion that had been created by the statement in Semmelweis's *Aetiology*, "After my departure on March 20, 1849 from the position of first assistant, **[67]** I petitioned for a private Docentur in obstetrics," which implied that Semmelweis had applied for his *habilitation* in the spring of 1849. 'Semmelweis's remark that his Docentur limited him to exercises on phantoms, which follows this passage, had also been used to construe this restriction as reflecting the personal rancor between Semmelweis and his opponents. However, the archival sources proved that the matter was much more complicated.'

'Two things (*Momente*) contradicted this interpretation of the restriction as being directed specifically against Semmelweis: first, the restriction reflected a fundamental question about "the *habilitation* requirements for demonstrative subjects;" second, the debate already involved another *habilitation* application, and led to its rejection on basic principles (*Erwägungen*). This was Zeissl's *habilitation* request, which, from February 1850 onwards, was so closely associated with Semmelweis's that this alone should have indicated that both proceedings involved the same principles. In fact, it is only from the history of Zeissl's *habilitation* that the events that made Semmelweis's *habilitation* application so precarious can be understood. Briefly, Zeissl's postdoctoral thesis involved the following issues:'

Zeissl was Hebra's student, and second physician on his department at the General Hospital, and on May 15, 1849 he had already sought conferment of a "Docentur for primary and 'consecutive' syphilis with use of affected patients on the Rash Division." He was able to get both management and Hebra to agree to this by appealing to a supplement specifically related to hospital management. However, Zeissl's application was rejected for technical reasons: because it failed to meet the new provisional habilitation standard issued on December 19, 1848 as almost all **[68]** the required supplements were missing—birth certificate, diploma, CV, even habilitation thesis. 'The fact that his application was nevertheless accepted (*weitergegeben wurde*) is a telling testimony of how transitional the year 1849 had been in Austrian university administration, saddled with all the uncertainties that the new legislation for university administrative practice brought with it.'

'On 29 December 1849, when Zeissl renewed his request with the necessary supplements, the end of his service as a second physician at the General Hospital (1st June 1850) was approaching. He submitted his application to Hebra for review, and on January 14, 1850, Hebra recommended that because Zeissl was not authorized to use any general hospital patients for demonstration purposes either during or after the expiration of his service as second physician, he should furnish the necessary teaching materials himself "from patients in his private practice, or from outpatient volunteers who agreed to be taught on." Although the College dropped Hebras's proposal at a meeting on January 19, 1850, and even recommended that Zeissl be *habilitated* without a lecture or a colloquium, but because the procurement of demonstrative materials in *habilitations* of this kind was posed by Zeissl's application, it was taken up by the Ministry; in its decree of February 17, 1850 concerning the *habilitation* of Dr. Zeissl, the Ministry asked the College of Professors whether "the Docentur requested by Dr. Zeissl should be regarded as a theoretical or a practical one, and if the latter case, what materials should be offered for practical instruction." The Ministry pointed out in the same decree "that the use of patients in the general hospital for educational purposes can only be done with the permission of the Ministry of Education ..."

This decree reached Dean Rokitansky on February 21, 1850, just as Semmelweis's *habilitation* was being processed, and it is a tragic irony that it should have been Hebra, Semmelweis's friend, who raised the question that was to cause so much grief to his friend. Rokitansky immediately recognized how dangerous the situation created by Zeissl's petition was for Semmelweis, **[69]** as from March 19, 1849 Semmelweis was no longer a member of the General Hospital. He sought to save the situation, and it is from that perspective that the previously mentioned supplement to Rokitansky's introduction to Semmelweis's application to the Ministry is to be understood: that enough "already otherwise-used corpses" would be available for exercises on cadavers. Nevertheless, the petitions of Semmelweis and Zeissl were both rejected on the same day, April 2, 1850: Semmelweis's on the grounds that "the use of cadavers for teaching by private docents was for several reasons impermissible;" Zeissl's with the remark that "private docentures on practical medicine can only be granted at the university if appropriate care is taken of the materials required for it:" Zeissl's proposal to use ambulatory patients from his private practice, and pictures and sculptural representations, for his lectures did not satisfy the Ministry.

'A monumental decision was made at the time of the decree of April 2 that was of vital importance to future Viennese clinicians: on 13

April 1850, it was decided that written objections were no longer to be sent to the Ministry of Education as Dean Rokitansky was authorized to speak in the name of the College of Professors to the Minister himself to explain the reasons the College determined that it was necessary for private Docents to use cadavers, as stated by the two candidates, Semmelweis and Zeissl.'

Lesky could not tell from the documentary material whether Rokitansky's audience with Thun came to pass and, if so, what success it had. But Semmelweis's friends were obviously convinced that a quick decision could not be expected given the meritorious nature of the question. Semmelweis and Zeissl, apparently on the advice **[70]** of Rokitansky and Skoda, 'did the right thing, considering the situation, and asked to be first granted a limited Docentur, which Semmelweis did on 9 May 1850, and Zeissl had already done on 26 April. Semmelweis's application had never been published before:'

> High Ministry of Education!
>
> After the high Ministry's decree complaining of the use of cadavers for teaching granted to private Docents became known to the reverent undersigned, the same permitted himself to express to the high ministry his willingness to limit his lectures on obstetrics to demonstrations on phantoms until the cadaver-question is definitively settled by the high Ministry, and therefore allows himself to repeat his most solemn request for the granting of a Docentur for theoretical obstetrics.
>
> *Vienna May 9, 1850*
>
> *Ig. Ph. Semmelweis*
> *Dr. der Medicin & Chirurgie*
> *Magister der Geburtshilfe*
> *Mitglied der medicin. Facultät,*
> *der Gesellschaft der Ärzte*
> *und emeritirte Assistenten der*
> *I. Gebärklinik zu Wien,*
> *Mitglied der Gesellschaft für*
> *Geburtshilfe u Berlin.*

'Semmelweis had signed all other documents merely with his name, but here he added all his degrees, titles, and memberships. His membership of the Society of Physicians in Vienna and of the Society for

Obstetrics in Berlin underscored what Rokitansky had emphasized to the Ministry in the introduction to Semmelweis's application: that Semmelweis's discovery was being increasingly recognized by experts.'

Semmelweis limited his request for a Docentur to exercises on the phantom. He had clearly assessed the situation **[71]** correctly, and that the restriction would only be an interim solution until "the cadaver question will have been definitively decided by a high ministry." The habilitation standard issued on 19 December 1848 was intentionally provisional in order to test it so that any gaps could be remedied in the definitive version. In the spring of 1850 the liveliest discussion of a new version had already started not only in the medical College of Professors, but also by the Philosophy faculty. A Ministerial Ordinance was already in print, and the new 1850 draft of the Habilitation of Private Docents, prepared on May 1, 1850 by the Philosophy Faculty, had already passed review by the well-known physiologist, Ernst Brücke. In Zeissl's case, Hebra had pointed out the need to supplement the provisions on demonstration material for habilitations in practical subjects. This was at a highly unfavorable time for Semmelweis, but given the attitude of the medical College of Professors under its Dean, Rokitansky, Semmelweis and Zeissl must have been confident that Rokitansky would find a solution favorable to them.

Rokotansky was not only Dean, but was at the same time an authoritative expert on the "cadaver question," and this was apparent from the attachment he presented to the Ministry of Education with Semmelweis and Zeissl's renewed habilitation application:

> High Ministry!
>
> The obedient undersigned presents to the high Ministry the renewed petitions of Messrs. Semmelweis and Zeissl, with the unanimous request of the College for their support.
>
> Dr. Semmelweis limited himself in his petition to a private Docentur on theoretical obstetrics as a consequence of the rejection of his request of February 9, which was motivated by the high ministerial decree of April 2, on the use of the phantom in his lectures.

[72] Dr. Zeissl, who the College of Professors found in its report of March 10, to be qualified to lecture on theoretical and practical syphilis, limits himself in his new request to theoretical lectures, and has presented a new program for this purpose.

With respect to the first, Dr. Semmelweis, the College allows itself once again to draw attention to the prowess recognized by experts, and to the great merit of his even more and more convincing discovery in the field of childbed fever; with respect to the latter, Dr. Zeissl, the College would like to support the modified application, in particular, because it believes that it would be better to give a qualified candidate a narrower scope than none at all.

In view of the instructions contained in the high decree of April 2 concerning the use of cadavers on the part of private Docents, the most obedient undersigned permits himself on behalf of the College to submit the following idea for consideration.

The need for cadavers, and cadaver parts for anatomy, physiology, for surgical, ophthalmological, and obstetrical surgical teachings and exercises, for the practical part of the pathological-anatomical and forensic lectures, is very great, and yet episodes of shortages of disposable corpses are not uncommon given the number of mortuaries. Only this deficiency affects different institutions very unequally, so unevenly that some are not aware of it. First, it is a delicate matter for those institutions that must have at their disposal an out-and-out unrestricted supply of cadavers, such as descriptive anatomy, and ophthlmological exercises. It is somewhat less delicate for surgical operative exercises in that urgent cases can be limited so that the mutilation of the face and hands is avoided. It is still less sensitive for physiology, which often addresses only a few body parts. It drops off for other subjects in that pathological and forensic dissections, and obstetrical operations can be done on any cadaver, because they do not mutilate cadavers intended for burial in a way that is perceptible to the public. Moreover, obstetrical, as well as ophthalmological and surgical lectures, can also use cadavers which were already the subject of a pathological or forensic autopsy.

In medicine, with the exception of a few subjects, the entire human corpse or its individual parts are such an indispensable teaching material that a fruitful duplication of lectures in a docentur cannot be imagined, if none of that teaching material can be offered.

[73] Now, admittedly, the need for corpses on the part of ordinary professors entitled to them is large, from time to time a noticeable lack could occur for one or the other, and if every docent was granted unlimited right to the purchase of corpses, the stock necessary for those teaching purposes could be unaffordable. But it is important to note that many specialties do not need entire copses, only individual parts, and many specialties are content with corpses that have already been used, and the former are also such that if necessary they can substitute animal parts for human cadaver parts.

On the basis of these discussions, the undersigned allows himself to ask the High Ministry in the name of the College, to make use of the cadavers available to Docents in so far as the need of the ordinary faculty permit. The High Ministry should, accordingly, grant the use of cadavers to all docents especially in specialties for which individual body parts or already used corpses suffice.

Vienna, March 17, 1850 *Rokitansky*
Dekan
Schroff

'The Ministry's decision came down on October 1, 1850. Since Schürer von Waldheim knew that the records in the Ministry of Education stated "exercises on phantoms and cadavers," he constructed a colorful assortment (*Strauß*) of hypotheses, conjectures, and speculations to connect the awarding of the Docentur to Semmelweis with his departure from Vienna a few days later. In the version "with exercises on the phantom and on cadavers," the Ministry would have, surprisingly, granted Semmelweis more than he had requested in his application of May 9, and would not explain why he left Vienna soon afterwards. So, Schürer came to the adventurous (*abenteuerlichen*) and unfounded view that the version of the *"Docentur* (*venia*)*"*[27] limited to use of phantoms that Semmelweis actually received involved fraud. Sinclair **[74]** took this up and ran with it: "The falsifier had no doubt gone to his own place long before Semmelweis had become of sufficient eminent [sic] in reputation to lead any one to investigate this final wrong in Vienna," he wrote.'

'Others thought that Semmelweis felt he was being hounded as a political rebel, or that he found the restriction on his Docentur an unbearable fresh humiliation by his enemies, Rosas and Klein. Schürer even went so far as to interpret Semmelweis's sudden decision to leave Vienna as signifying brain disease. Whichever hypotheses one chooses, the almost universal conviction has been that there was a causal connection between the disappointment of being awarded a limited Docentur and Semmelweis's sudden departure from Vienna. For one can thank ["invoke"] the most used Semmelweis biographer: Semmelweis himself. After describing the Docentur that he had been awarded, Semmelweis stated, "In the month of October, 1850, I moved to my native city, Pest" but by prefixing it with the word "therefore," he converted a declarative sentence into a 'conclusion.' Only Isador Fischer had questioned the fraud version spread (*in die Welt gesetzten*) by Schüer, and stated that in Schürer's explanation of "with exercises on phantoms and cadavers" one sentence was valid: "The matter requires clarification."'

What actually happened is revealed by the draft of the relevant decree that was attached to Semmelweis's application of May 9, signed by hand, and also endorsed by Exner, the ministerial advisor in the Ministry of Education and co-creator of the Thun-Hohenstein reform, and which has the following wording:

> Through the consistory of the University of Vienna to the College of Medical Professors:

[27] 'venia' is short for venia legend (permission to read) bestowed after a habilitation candidate has delivered his or her public lecture following the acceptance of the candidate's habilitation thesis.

[75] The Ministry of Culture and Education grants Dr. Ignaz Semmelweis's request for a private Docentur in theoretical obstetrics limited to practice and exercises on phantoms, and Dr. Hermann Zeissl's request for a private Docentur of syphilis with the restriction that he only uses pictures of the preparations in the pathology museum in his private lectures.

Herewith N. N. completes its report of May 17 (d. J. Z. 637), with reference to the supplements to be returned to Drs. Semmelweis and Zeissl, with the advice that the question concerning the authorization of the use of cadavers in lessons taught by private students is to be dealt with separately.

Gas. Ex. *Well*

This document clarified and brought an end to the docentur question by establishing conclusively that the docentur granted to Semmelweis by the Ministry of Education was limited to demonstrations on exercises on phantoms, and provides no support for Schürer's fraud hypothesis and Sinclair's subsequent supposition.

'An even more meaningful conclusion could be drawn from what Well had added to the end of the draft [of the docentur decree], and from the changes that this addition subsequently underwent: that the medical College of Professors obviously wanted to put off deciding the cadaver-question to a later time.'

'Well chose a wording that left nothing to be desired in terms of its vagueness and ambiguity. Only the heading of Well's text of the question under discussion, "Use of cadavers in lessons taught by private Docents," was retained. Thun-Hohenstein had himself used this heading, the same minister who, by his last-minute, personal intervention, prevented the departure of the excellent oculist, Ferdinand Arlt, from Prague to Leipzig in 1849, and who brought the internist Johann Oppolzer, who had already emigrated to Leipzig, back to Austria, and who, **[76]** as we know from unpublished letters, was so valued by the scientifically-minded Ernst Wilhelm Brücke, that he made his stay in Vienna dependent on Thun remaining in office. This Minister personally crossed out Well's proposal, and attached the following new instruction with his signature, "Exp Th.""

> Concerning the use of cadavers for teaching by private Docents, N.N. is requested to consider the circumstances, and to give a reasoned opinion in each individual case as to whether and under what restrictions, if any, Docents should be granted such use.
>
> *Exp. Th.*

Thun took Rokitansky's express reference to the cadaver-question in the report that on March 17, 1850 Rokitansky attached to the Act, and in which Rokitansky recommended that the Ministry 'grant the use of cadavers to all docents in specialties in which use of individual body parts or already-used cadavers suffice.' He was trying to secure a positive decision on the cadaver-question, and intended the wording of his supplement to leave open the possibility for the College to revisit the question or by emphasizing the word "grant" at the end of his supplement, was inviting it to do so.

'One goes astray if, unaware of the archival sources, one interprets the award of a limited docentur to Semmelweis as signifying a new humiliating act of malice set in motion by his old enemies, Rosas and Klein, because the docentur—however small and limited it may have been—was the first tangible success in the great struggle that the Rokitansky-Skoda School had achieved in a nearly two-year, hard struggle for Semmelweis. Its first success against the Ministry!' The earlier victory that the school had already achieved on 15 May 1850, was 'against their and Semmelweis's enemy, against Semmelweis himself. That is how long it took until Semmelweis [77] felt ready to accede to the wishes of his friends, to the request of the Society of Physicians on February 23, 1849, and speak for the first time about his discovery.' Semmelweis had given his lecture on 15 May 1850, between the time he submitted his second petition (on 9 May) and Rokitansky forwarded it to the Ministry (on 17 May), and only under great pressure, 'after the account which his teacher, Skoda, had given of his discovery with his Academy lecture had been violently attacked by Scanzoni from Prague.'

‘This lecture by Semmelweis on 15 May was the first major success of the Viennese school in its fight for Semmelweis. It has entered the annals of the Society of Physicians as a “true triumph of research.” In October, it was joined by another success with the implementation of his Docentur. The possibility of expanding the limited Docentur already loomed. No doubt: despite all the difficulties, Rokitansky and Skoda had finally managed to give the career of their student a gratifying turn. At this point, in mid-October, the incomprehensible occured: Semmelweis escaped from Vienna. He later probably felt he had to justify it, and sought to do it in his main work with the words: “I could not use such a limited Docentur as for a qualification obtained from a Docent to be valid, the scope of the instruction had to be the same as that from a professor, but professors were at liberty to conduct demonstrations and exercises on cadavers as well.”’

Semmelweis refers quite correctly here to the Ministerial Decree “on the position, duties and rights of private-docents in educational institutions, which enjoy the freedom to teach and learn.” It has the following wording:

> The private docents ... are entitled to issue certificates of attendance and progress... **[78]** These certificates have the same legal effect as those provided by professors who teach obligatory subjects, provided that the lectures of the private docents are the same in purpose and scope as those of the professors.

‘Semmelweis’s docentur, which was limited to demonstrations on phantoms, did not meet the decree’s requirements to issue certificates. But this decree was issued on January 5, 1849, and Semmelweis must have known about it long before May 9, 1850, when “expressed his readiness to restrict his lectures to demonstrations on phantoms.” Therefore, there can be no question about the restriction on the Docentur coming as a surprise. He was granted the Docentur on October 1, 1850 that he had applied for on May 9, 1850. The October 1 decree of appointment contains no new facts Semmelweis would not have known about at the filing on May 9, except for the above-mentioned addition of the Minister whose significance was more likely to be favourable for Semmelweis. If one combines these facts in the newly discovered documents with Semmelweis's attempt to justify his sudden departure from Vienna in mid-October with the restriction on his docentur, one cannot help but diagnose that this attempt represents a later self-interpretation. Here Semmelweis's case stops being historical and starts to become more psychological.'

Appointment to Pest Faculty

Before opening the last chapter of the Vienna School's fight for Semmelweis, one has to look to Budapest, and 'note with all soberness that even Semmelweis's home was not at first ready to offer the country's great son the position which his achievement should have secured him.' There were, at that time, two Obstetric-Gynecological services in Pest: the maternity ward at St. Rochus Hospital, a municipal institution with one ward and two maternity rooms, and a state-owned university maternity hospital. Semmelweis became the "unpaid honorary director" of the first institution until May 20, 1851, **[79]** which meant that he was allowed to work there unpaid, and practice his prophylaxis of puerperal fever. He did that with great success. Semmelweis's career took a new turn in 1855, when the Professor of Obstetrics position at the University of Pest became vacant after the death of Florian Birly. The manner in which this position was filled is so full of hitherto unknown, illuminating details that it deserves to be taken note of. The illuminating details of how this post was filled are contained in a recitation of the Education Minister, Count Leo Thun von Hohenstein in the administrative archives, to which the reports of the Civil and Military administrations for Hungary, as well as on the bureau of the Lieutenancy in Ofen, were attached.'

Semmelweis was not the Pest medical faculty's first choice: it was Carl Braun. Semmelweis was in second place, and Franz Valla was in third place. 'The votes for first place were: four votes for Braun, one vote for Semmelweis, one vote for Valla; the votes for second place were: one vote for Braun, three votes for Semmelweis, one vote for, Valla; and the votes for third place were: three votes for Semmelweis, four votes for Valla.'

There were seven applicants for the post, and they were ranked in a Competence table according to certain criteria (duration of prior appointment, language skills) pursuant to an old Austrian administrative practice. One was added to the usual criteria related to the events of 1848, with the question "cleared by the imperial military court?" that today would be understood to mean 'political behavior.' The answer for Semmelweis was "he was an Assistant during the revolutionary turmoil in Vienna." The certificate of clearance from the Mayor's office in Pest regarding Semmelweis's political and 'moral' behavior during his sojourn prior to February 12, 1851 **[80]** was no longer in the file, 'but a presentation to the Kaiser indicates that it was favorable and, based on this assessment, one can infer that Semmelweis was politically unobjectionable and had committed no offenses in the years 1851-1855, and conclude the same about the time of his assistantship in Vienna.'

'It is true that Schürer von Waldheim always liked to point out that Semmelweis was a member of the Academic Legion in March 1848, and was one of the "most enthusiastic, most ardent freedom fighters." However, that does not mean he would have been politically compromised. Many of Semmelweis's colleagues and teachers, such as Hebra and Hyrtl, belonged to the Academic Legion in the spring of 1848, and were acknowledged and permitted to function as security guards by an imperial decree. The situation only changed after the October Revolution of 1848. Membership of the Academic Legion was then banned and considered incriminating. If Semmelweis had not taken into account the political situation at that time, as, for example, his friend, Georg Maria Lautner, had not and was arrested, it would have been easy for Rosas and Klein to reject Semmelweis's request for an extension of his assistantship for this reason alone. But since both of them had to work in a most sophisticated way with the old and new regulations in order to justify refusing his request for an extension, one may conclude, *ex silencio*, that Semmelweis did not participate in the struggle for freedom in 1848 beyond what was allowed by the government.'

Another question could be clarified from the fact that the Competency Table indicated that Semmelweis lectured in Hungarian, which had often been cited to prove that Semmelweis was Hungarian. But Lesky had never doubted 'Semmelweis's Magyar national feelings,' only noted that this could not be inferred from the fact that he lecture in Hungarian.

'Since the beginning of the 19th century, the Austrian education administration, especially when it came to the appointment of surgical and obstetrical professorships in parts of the country that spoke foreign languages, had been strict about appointing docents who spoke the national language. Given the same professional qualifications, **[81]** candidates who had the appropriate language skills used to be favored. This principle was based on the eighteenth century idea that greatest wealth of a state was in having as large and as healthy a population as possible. As regards populations, having good country surgeons and good midwives was the first requirement of good medical policy, which Johann Peter Frank and the *Protomedicus* of the Hereditary Lands, Joseph Andreas von Stifft, tried to implement as advisors to the Court Chancellery and the study Court Commission. But how could good midwives be educated in the different parts of the multiethnic state where different languages were spoken, if their teachers could not teach them new obstetrical knowledge in their native tongue? So, by the beginning of the nineteenth century the principle had emerged that, when filling vacant teaching positions, the first requirement was to know the relevant national language. Boer's former assistant, Florian Birly (1787-1855), Semmelweis's predecessor as professor in Pest, had also given lectures in Hungarian. The files specifically emphasized that he appropriated this "idiom" to such an extent "that he was able to make himself very understandable to the midwives." In addition to the fact that Semmelweis continued Birly's tradition of lecturing in Hungarian, his official correspondence was also in Hungarian.'

'It has so far been overlooked that in the old monarchy, which people liked to refer to as a "multiethnic dungeon," there was a separate language decree for clinical chairpersons. The High Commission for Studies had passed it in September 1841, and it extended beyond obstetrical and surgical areas to all professorial appointments in the entire medial field. This decree specified that "every time applications for a professorship are announced, the ability to speak the vernacular of the country in which the professorship is held, will be made an express requirement." That is why Semmelwes's as well as Franz Hektor von Arneth's applications for Professor of Obstetrics **[82]** in Prague (1851) had to be rejected as neither of them spoke Czech. Therefore, it was all the more astonishing to learn from the Ministry how the Pest medical faculty applied the language principle in selecting the professor of obstetrics, as it gave Carl Brown, who had little prior knowledge of Hungarian, preference over Semmelweis.'

'Apparently, the Pest faculty was guided in its decision by the fact that Carl Braun had already published "Clinical Obstetrics and Gynecology" (issued in 1855) with his colleagues, Johann Baptist Chiari and Joseph Späth, a work which its review suggested was received "with very acclaimed criticism" at home and abroad. However, as of 1855, Semmelweis had not written a line. Nevertheless, the higher administrative authorities, the bureau of Lieutenancy in Ofen and the Civil and Military Administration of Hungary in Vienna, held fast to the principle of the language qualification requirement for the teaching staff. And, of course, this was done by the Ministry of Education in Vienna, the successor to the student High Commission, which had issued the language decree of 1841. This Ministry, which was so outspokenly opposed to the extension of Semmelweis's assistantship, now gave, over and above his language qualification, such a tribute to his achievements that it deserves to be recorded here word for word:'

> The professor of obstetrics at the University of Pest cannot dispense with knowledge of Hungarian. Waiting for a professor who does not know this language to acquire it appropriately, and give indispensable assistance to the education of midwives, cannot be justified in the present case where the Chief physician, Dr. Semmelweis has all the qualities for the professorship to a high degree.
>
> During his employment as Assistant in obstetrics at the University of Vienna, Dr. Semmelweiss gave brilliant proof of his talent, his love of obstetrics, his untiring zeal in the learning and perfecting this subject, and worked on the scientific side of it with **[83]** just as much ingenuity and thoroughness, as technical skill and good luck. His views on the origin and spread of puerperal fever, as well

as on the means of preventing or curbing it, are not without scientific and practical foundations, and have been recognized by the most capable of obstetricians.

His lectures as Assistant and private docent of Obstetrics in Vienna were characterized by their scientific value and liveliness, and were well attended. His service as Chief of Obstetrics at Rochus Hospital is likewise described as a very beneficial one. Since this candidate is sufficiently proficient in Hungarian, and reports on his moral and political conduct are favorable, it cannot be disputed that the State division of the Ofen Bureau and the Civil and Military Administration of Hungary have deemed Dr. Semmelweis the most suitable of the applicants for the teaching position.

Therefore, I would like to make the most humble request: that Your Majesty graciously accede that Dr. Ignaz Semmelweis, Chief Physician at St. Rochus Hospital, be appointed professor in theoretical and practical obstetrics at the University of Pest with the salary of one thousand three hundred gulden CM, and the rights of advancement in the higher salary grades of 1600fl and 1900 fl.

Vienna, July 4, 1855 *Helfert*
For the Minister
Undersecretary of State

'The fact that this request was signed by Undersecretary Helfert, the same man who had caused Semmelweis such difficulties six years earlier together with Rosas and Klein, shows what a drastic change took place within Austria's highest teaching authority towards Semmelweis during the Thun era. On July 18, 1855, he was appointed professor of obstetrics in Pest. On 1 April 1856 Klein died in Vienna. Why should Semmelweis not be his successor? The fundamentally changed attitude of the ministry could well justify this hope.'

Klein's Succession (1856)

A notice in the Viennese Medical Weekly **[84]** on 2 August 1856 stated that on August 1st the Viennese medical College of Professors proposed for appointment as Professor of Obstetrics, 'Carl Braun from Trient in first place, Joseph Späth, supernumerary Professor at the Joseph Acadamy, in second place, and Eduard Lumpe in third place. Schürer von Waldheim unearthed this note, and commented on it as follows:'

> "That Semmelweis was not only not proposed in first place, but not at all, was the rather personal, ignoble response of the Viennese College of Professors to Semmelweis's foolishness of October 1850. He had thrown the docentur at their feet; one does not want to expose oneself to such treatment a second time... Such a renunciation, such a superior attitude from the College of Professors, from Skoda, should not have been expected. Skoda was only human too."

'It is high time to set against these baseless claims the historical facts revealed by the files still preserved in the Administrative and University Archives. Although they confirm the above sequence as correct, a radical correction of Schürer's claim is nevertheless necessary. The Appointments Committee of the Vienna Medical Faculty, fully aware of its responsibility to make an apt decision, dealt in great detail with Semmelweis's performance. After all, the members of this committee, as advisors, were Bartsch, professor of the midwives division, the surgeon Shuh, and Semmelweis's old friend and comrade, Theodor Helm, who had protested so vigorously in 1849 against Braun's appointment as Assistant.'

Semmelweis had not actually applied for the position, and the Appointments Committee had itself increased the number of applicants by bringing in obstetricians from both inside and outside Austria, and of these (Benrhard Seyfert, Prague, Johann Streng, Prague, **[85]** Franz Hektor von Arneth, St. Petersbug, Friedrick Wilhelm Scanzoni, Würzburg , Wilhelm Lange, Heidelberg, Franz Breit, Tübingen), Semmelweis was the first to be asked. But in evaluating their individual accomplishments, the Appointments Committee emphasized the following: 'Members of the committee are in agreement over their proposal that, in addition to knowledge of their scientific field and teaching ability... it should also take into consideration existing literary achievements in particular as also a means of promoting science, namely, ascertain the current status of their lessons as this must be regarded as the task of professors.'

'One can see that the Appointments Committee of the Viennese faculty, by making literary achievement a criterion, was guided by the same point of view as the Pest faculty the previous year. But nine years after his discovery, Semmelweis had not published a single line on this or any other subject in his field. Here it becomes completely clear how disastrous Semmelweis's reluctance to publish was for his career, as well as the dissemination of his doctrine. Indeed, his assistant, Joseph Fleischer, had published "A statistical report from the Imperial University of Pest for the year 1855-56" in the August 16, 1856 issue of the Viennese Medical Journal, and pointed out the renewed success of chlorine washings, as Hebra, Skoda, Haller, and Arneth had done. But even this report could at best only be a reminder of his achievement, which, incidentally, it did not need, because three weeks before the publication of this report, the Appointments Committee had in its recommendation of July 16, 1856, already commented that Semmelweis's achievement was extremely commendable (*ausserordentlich ehrenvoll*):'

> As far as the additional qualification and teaching ability are concerned, the committee finds itself prompted here to mention in particular Professor Semmelweis, who, as Assistant (in the years 1847-48-49 and Acc. Docent 1849), received full approval and support from many thoughtful investigators for his view of the origin of puerperal diseases, especially through cadaverous infection, and indisputably threw a new light **[86]** on the development of these diseases, and thereby, as well as by a statistical compilation of puerperal diseases in the various maternity hospitals of the monarchy, gained real merit; however, recognizing this merit, the members of the committee must all the more regret that Professor Semmelweis has not published in his field during these last few years, which literary works it would have like to point to, and to have seen follow his otherwise eminent skills.

'These considerations led to the above-mentioned recommendation on 16 July 1856. Then something astonishing happened on the 27th of July: a group of professors joined in a separate recommendation [*Separatvotum*], and placed that man in first place from whom there was not one printed line, who “threw the lectureship at the feet of the Viennese professors six years ago,” and who a year ago the medical faculty of his hometown had relegated to the second place. This memorable separate recommendation, in which the old Viennese professors and friends of Semmelweis acknowledged him again and thereby made known the complete scientific achievement in a personal way across space and time, bears next to it the names of Rokitansky and Dlauhy, as well as Skoda, whose generosity Schürer so underestimated. But that’s not enough! Another must also have his rights against the recklessness of this accepted fable.’

‘This separate recommendation was drafted by the surgeon Dumreicher, who, according to Schürer, was completely unaffected by Semmelweis’s discovery because he was “without a higher view of the whole.” In truth, however, Dumreicher leached dressings in chlorine lime solution for days, and wound care on his clinic was so **[87]** meticulously clean that in thirty years his clinic was visited only twice by the bugaboo of all surgical wards: hospital infections, a telling contrast to other surgical clinics where up to 80% of amputees died of hospital infections in the pre-antiseptic period. When in 1861, Semmelweis explained in his main work that “my doctrine is not forgotten at the school from where it originated,” this was true, above all, of Dumreicher, who had applied it on the first surgical clinic with success.’

‘So it is understandable that Dumreicher stood up for Semmelweis from the very beginning. In 1849 Skoda had borne the brunt of the fight, in 1850 it had fallen to Rokitansky as the then Dean, so now in 1856 it was the surgeon, Dummreicher, who seized the initiative in the appointment-question with great inner élan in his separate vote:’

> After the result of the vote on the appointment of the Professor of Obstetrics, the high Ministry was deprived of the views of the minority of the College Professors, the undersigned feel obliged to intervene in the interest of education and science, and present its opinion and separate vote to the high Ministry:
>
> The undersigned are convinced that Professor Semmelweis deserves to be considered among the domestic applicants for appointment, and base their opinion on the following:

1. A High Ministry appointed Professor Semmelweis to the position of Professor of Obstetrics at the University of Pest, the candidate now proposed in first place for the Professorship in Vienna. Since the appointment of Professor Semmelweis, the circumstances have changed only in as much as through his work he has completely **[88]** justified the confidence placed in him by a High Ministry, is respected by his colleagues, admired by his hearers, has earned the public's full confidence, and is justly considered one of the most outstanding professors at the University of Pest.

2. In filling this chair at the University of Vienna, it seems desirable to take into account the general medical-scientific education of the applicant, also consider specialized knowledge, not only in the narrower field of obstetrics, but also of female genital diseases generally.

Professor Semmelweis's tireless and successful quest to develop this area (*Zweige*) is apparent from the fact that over a three year period he performed manual examinations for research purposes of the female genital organs of all female cadavers in the mortuary of the Imperial General Hospital, and attended the autopsies if he found any abnormalities. Through this research and study, which required uncommon sacrifice, he had, after one year, obtained results for diagnosing these diseases, and that Prof. Chiari, who sadly for science, died too early, and Dr. Arneth, who had arranged them, continued these examinations with Dr. Semmelweis for two years, so that one can rightly claim that the more precise diagnosis of these diseases had essentially been stimulated and encouraged in Vienna by Dr. Semmelweis, and there would hardly be a gynecologist who had gained more knowledge and experience in diagnosing these diseases.

3. The facts are clear that during the two years that Dr. Semmelweis worked as Assistant at the local maternity clinic, the disastrous puerperal epidemic that killed thousands of human lives in our and other maternity hospitals, and that in no year spared our

institution, completely disappeared, and that while he worked in his institution in Pest, the mortality percentage was also reduced to a minimum.

Professor Semmelweis believes that certain, appropriate, strictly-enforced measures can prevent this epidemic in maternity hospitals, and many lives could be saved. The honorable Professor Chiari, who was proficient in his field, and a relative of Professor Klein who opposed Dr. Semmelweis's views, embraced Dr. Semmelweis's view, and sought to prove it with lectures and scientific articles about his experience. From other **[89]** sides, the correctness of this assumption was contradicted.

The resolution of this controversy is of the highest human and scientific importance to doctors and philanthropists. No institution is in such a position to decide this important controversy as our University. If, however, this question is to be decided, then the definite measures must be strictly enforced through a number of years, and the facts will then decide. It is in the nature of things, and only human, that one who is opposed to a point of view, or who does not share a conviction, will institute, perform, and oversee measures for years with less zeal, with less care and accuracy than the man who, having prevented puerperal epidemic in Europe's largest institution for two years, is convinced of it.

The undersigned are convinced, and are justified in believing, that Dr. Semmelweis is overall most qualified and worthy to represent this teaching institution; the decision of the said important issue for science and every philanthropist makes his appointment from this point of view also appear desirable.

Vienna, July 27, 1856 — *Professor v. Dumreicher*

In complete agreement with this view — *Prof. Dlauthy*, *Prof. Skoda*

Whose presence at the meeting was prevented by illness — *Prof. Rokitansky*

'Dumreicher skilfully reminds the Ministry at the beginning of his recommendation that Semmelweis had been appointed professor in Pest, and that during his first year of clinical activity Semmelweis had fully justified the Ministry's confidence in him. He also recalled the success with which Semmelweis had worked in Vienna. Here, the old concern of Skoda and the reform group with proving the value of the Semmelweis discovery beyond all doubt comes to the fore as the strongest argument and most urgent consideration from a scientific and philanthropic viewpoint. This memorandum refuted Schürer's **[90]** claim that this Viennese surgeon was "without a higher view of the whole" because Dumreicher considered Semmelweis to be the most suitable candidate by reason of his "general medical education" and "special knowledge, not only of the narrow field of obstetrics, but also of diseases of the female genitalia in general." The apt remarks in this sentence shed new light on Semmelweis and Gynecology. Indeed, one had already known—as Semmelweis had himself said— that since 1944 he had been particularly fond of the new subject of gynaecology, and that he was a self-made man in this field as for six years he "dissected practically every day all the female cadavers" in Rokitansky's morgue. But it has not been asked what meaning and significance Semmelweis's gynaecological post-mortems had at the time in the context of his school.'

'The answer can only be that with his autopsy work in the field of gynecology Semmelweis fulfilled the Rokitansky school's very own concern with substantiating clinical diagnoses anatomico-pathologically in order to obtain an precise basis from the autopsy table for clinical gynecological diagnoses. Skoda did the same thing for internal medicine, Hebra for dermatology, Bednar for paediatrics, Stellwag von Carion for ophthalmology and Shuh for surgery. By checking their bedside findings at the autopsy table, all these clinicians sought to fulfil the Rokitansky School's primary concern for precise clinico-anatomical correlations. But while each of these clinicians could make their correlations by first collecting evidence from the living in their respective clinical wards, and then correlating their findings with Rokitansky's dissections, Semmelweis was denied this opportunity, and so in this context, Semmelweis's rueful statement that "it was not possible for me to study Gynecology that is so necessary for an obstetrician at the Imperial **[91]** general hospital," deserves finally to be taken seriously. This statement needs clarification, but it can be clarified only by recalling the local circumstances, that is, by briefly surveying the state of gynecological research in Vienna in the early 1840s.'

'There had, in fact, been a gynecological department at the General Hospital since 1843. However, it was not associated with either the first or the second maternity division, which were dedicated to making their clinical material freely available for teaching and research. Rather, this gynecological department was affiliated with the so-called private wing (*Zahlabteilung*) of the hospital, which was a separate department from the maternity divisions (founded in 1784) and was always headed by its own separate chief, which, since 1842 (sic), had been Eduard Mikschik (1809-1856). In 1851, Franz Hektor von Arneth reported that at that time this private wing still had strictly to follow the provisions on patient confidentiality made at the time by Joseph II with the best philanthropic intent. In 1843 Eduard Mikschik established this gynecological department, consisting of two hospital rooms, that Semmelweis spoke about in the passage quoted earlier. So, Semmelweis's comment is to be understood as that even "as an aspirant for the assistant position on the first maternity division, later as a provisional and finally as the actually assistant on this division" ... Semmelweis was not able to study on the gynecological division of the imperial general hospital.'

'It only bears witness again to Semmelweis's unwaveringly inquiring mind that even in this hopeless situation, he knew how to create a 'surrogate' (*Ersatz*) for the clinical observations he lacked. He found it in Rokitansky's autopsy room. The women who had died on the gynecological department also went there. There, as we learned from Dumreicher's separate vote and from him (Semmelweis) himself, he carried out manual examinations of dead women that he could not carry out in the living. Since the field of gynecology mainly involved tactile findings, and not, as in the Skoda's case, auditory findings, **[92]** the post-mortem examination could in fact replace a clinical one to some extent. In as much as he immediately checked his manual findings with the autopsy findings, and fulfilled to a great extent the anatomico-clinical concern of the Rokitansky-Skoda school in the field of gynecology, we can only now get a proper understanding of what Dumreicher had written in his separate vote: Semmelweis became a pioneer of gynecological diagnosis in Vienna. What is particularly surprising to learn is that Semmelweis, who was a former pupil of Klein's former assistant in obstetrics, Johann Baptist von Chiari (1817-1854), was, in gynecology, his and his colleague's, Franz Hector von Arneth's, teacher. It is this Chiari who, after Semmelweiss's lecture in the great debate at the Medical Society on July 15, 1850, unambiguously acknowledged Semmelweis's doctrine in his essay, "Tips for preventing puerperal epidemics," as well as Arneth, who in 1851 familiarized his French and English colleagues in Paris and Edinburgh with this doctrine, and in 1860 was able to convert his colleagues in St. Petersburg. But while the gynecological achievements of these two Viennese physicians, especially the Chiaris, have gained a firm place in the history of the Viennese school, all the pioneering work in gynecology that Semmelweis carried out in Rokitansky's autopsy room remained unknown until now.'

'Here the deeply rooted problem in Semmelweis's nature and personality, which had such a fatal effect on his academic career, shows itself again. While Chiari, who Semmelweis inspired, and who became Mirschik's successor in the private wing of the maternity hospital in 1847, had his "Gynecological Contributions" ready for printing 1852, Semmelweis could not bring himself to publish the slightest amount until 1857. When Dumreicher, Rokitansky, Skoda, and Dlauhy **[93]** submitted their separate vote to the faculty on July 27, 1856, there was not a printed line by Semmelweis. It was precisely this fact that left only these four stalwart fighters for Semmelweis. On 16 November 1856 Carl Braun was appointed Klein's successor. The fight for Semmelweis had thus come to an end. But the four signatories of the separate vote, among them the two leaders of the second Viennese Medical School, Rokitansky and Skoda, to their great credit, stayed in this nine-year struggle, recognized the genius of the man despite all the problems associated with his nature, and, accordingly, acted tenaciously.'

CRITIQUE

The central question Lesky's monograph sought to answer was what Semmelweis's discovery of the cause and prophylaxis of childbed fever owed to the Vienna Medical School. The available historical evidence established that it was all the materials necessary to make Semmelweis's discovery possible—(1) an almost unlimited supply of cadavers, (C&C, 13); (2) unfettered access to all female cadavers, (Lesky, 185); (3) two maternity divisions to which patients were admitted on alternate days, i.e. almost on a random basis, (SM, 355-356); and (4) records of monthly maternal mortality rates for the lying-in hospital, and for each maternity division, going back to the founding of the AKH in 1784. (SM, 398, Table XVII) To this must be added the concept of disease as a process rather than a state that Rokitansky imparted to Semmelweis and the Vienna Medical School, and which was the only intellectual link between Semmelweis discovery and that school.

All this was known by the time Lesky wrote her monograph but she was not content with the answer because, as she herself acknowledged, that would reduce the Vienna Medical School's contribution to what she considered to be 'one of the greatest discoveries in the history of medicine' to merely correlating the clinical signs and symptoms of disease with the underlying pathological changes, [**M, 57**]—and there was nothing new in that (see below). Everything that the Vienna Medical School supplied was clearly insufficient to elucidate why the MMR on the first division was three times higher than on the second, because none of the many commissions appointed to elucidate the reason was able to find the answer. For that, something more was required: what Owen Wangensteen characterized as a "penetrating insight without parallel in the history of medicine."[28] That insight belonged to Semmelweis alone, and owed little to the Vienna Medical School and even less to Skoda. Benedek summed

---

[28] Wangensteen, p. 566.

the situation up aptly, and, with the caveat that an attenuated link did exist between that insight and Rokitansky's concept of disease, justly:

> 'The Vienna Medical School was outstanding, but could never rise to the required level when it came to the question of childbed fever. Semmelweis indeed learned a lot from Rokitansky and from Skoda, but as to the discovery of childbed fever, these two great men played no part whatsoever.' (B, 87)

Lesky portrayed Semmelweis as having a special, 'intimate' student-teacher relationship with Skoda, and as most wanting to be his assistant to support what has been the enduring legacy of her narrative: the fallacy that Semmelweis made his discovery by applying the methodology he learned from Skoda, which Lesky referred to as the *'per exclusionem'* method or 'disjunctive syllogism, *modus tollendo ponens.*' It is true that Semmelweis attended Skoda's lectures, and he did apply to be Skoda's assistant, but this was not his first choice, as Lesky herself acknowledged the following year in her *magnum opus* about the Vienna Medical School:

> 'Bednar, together with Semmelweis, who was two years his junior, and Stellwag, belonged to a group of students who gathered around Rokitansky and his assistant Jakob Kolletschka (1803-1847) in a particularly intimate circle...he and Semmelweis applied simultaneously for the position of assistant to Kolletschka. Both were unsuccessful... Semmelweis, before finally deciding on obstetrics in 1846, made one other application, this time for the position of assistant to Skoda.' (Lesky, 141).

The special relationship that Lesky claimed existed between Semmelweis and Skoda actually existed between Semmelweis and Rokitansky and other pathologists in Rokitansky's department, not Skoda. Indeed, the pathologists were the only members of the AKH about whom Semmelweis made positive comments in his *Aetiology*, writing that he was "able to boast of Rokitansky's friendship," (SM, 405) and "revered" Kolletschka "highly," (SM, 391), and calling Lautner his friend. (SM, 409) Semmelweis never wrote a negative word about any of his teachers in his *Aetiology*, not even Klein. The only exception was Skoda, who,

Semmelweis ruefully noted, 'mentioned some things not pertaining to childbed fever' in his lecture to the Academy of Sciences. (SM, 609).

After graduating as a physician in April, 1844, Semmelweis spent much of the next two years before becoming Klein's assistant performing autopsies in Rokitansky's morgue on all mothers who had died of childbed fever, and on their babies if they had also died after birth, which was often the case. He also examined and dissected female cadavers who had died of gynaecological diseases to teach himself gynecology, as gynecology was part of the private wing [*Zahlabteilung*], not the maternity divisions of the AKH, and not taught to medical students. [**M, 91**]. Lesky acknowledged that '[t]he fact that in 1844 Rokitansky made available to him all female cadavers at the pathological institute was undoubtedly of great importance to Semmelweis.' (Lesky, 185), and that Semmelweis became 'a pioneer of gynecological diagnoses in Vienna,' and the teacher of his former teachers, Chiari and Arneth, in gynecology. [**M, 92**] Astonishingly, even after he became the Klein's assistant, Semmelweis began his workday by performing autopsies on women who had died of childbed fever the previous day, before examining all in-patients in preparation for Klein's morning ward rounds. (SM, 406).

Thus, Semmelweis developed considerable expertise in gross pathology, and was well placed to make the anatomico-pathological correlations on which his deduction about the cause of childbed fever was based when Semmelweis said he made them, refuting Podach's contrary conclusion that Lesky endorsed (see below). Lesky did refer to "pathological-anatomical precondition" as being a component of Semmelweis's theory, but never explained what she meant by it:

> 'Once we consider this discovery in terms of its methodological constituents, we can highlight three prongs: 1. The pathological-anatomical precondition; 2. A very specific final comparative-analytic procedure, which Sinclair characterized well as 'Elimination of Factors,' and 3. crowning it all, the statistical proof… But Semmelweis was also able to combine what he recognized morphologically into an etiological and clinical entity. In this tripartite correlation, the correctness of the Rokitansky-Skoda school received its broadest support in Semmelweis's discovery.' [**M, 56-57**]

No one can fairly claim to know what all this meant except that by 'pathological-anatomical precondition' Lesky could not have been referring to Semmelweis's actual pathological reasoning for she rejected Semmelweis's own account of his discovery (see below). But she was perfectly clear about how she contended Semmelweis deduced the cause of childbed: he simply excluded all the putative causes of childbed fever by applying Skoda's *per exclusionem* method until only one possibility was left: infection introduced into the birth canals of labouring women by the contaminated fingers of their attendants who had been involved in autopsies, since only students were taught on the first division, and only they were involved in autopsies, not midwives. That was all there was to it:

> 'This eerie difference had troubled the heads of governmental commissions, and raised hypotheses upon hypotheses: weather influences, the genius epidemicus in particular; overcrowding and bad ventilation of the rooms, their year-long infection with "puerperal miasma;" the anxiety of the newly delivered on the deadly first maternity division; clinic; yes, even the wounded feeling of shame of women at being examined by students, and, above all, the medical treatment on this division were all to blame for this gruesome difference in mortality. Skoda's student, Semmelweis, thinned this jungle of fictitious etiologies by exercising the method of exclusion he learned from his master. He distinguished one possibility listed above after the other, and in a comparative analysis he checked specifically whether the factors cited were able to account for the difference in mortality in a satisfactory, that is to say scientifically based way. Finally, there was only one option left: infection of the birth parts (*Geburtsteile*) by cadaveric-poison on the unwashed fingers of doctors and students.' **[M, 58-59]**

This was not only an incorrect account of Semmelweis's reasoning, it was not even an accurate account of Skoda's description of Semmelweis's discovery not the least because Skoda did give a pathological basis for Semmelweis's reasoning (albeint not the correct one), and Skoda did not enumerate all the factors Semmelweis had excluded.

The *'per exclusionem'* method simply referred to a diagnosis of exclusion, i.e. diagnoses based not on the affirmative signs and symptoms present but on excluding all known potential causes of the symptoms and signs in question. Self-evidently, exclusion of known potential causes cannot without more elucidate an as yet unknown cause of a disease, nor was it ever designed to do so. The same is true of the disjunctive syllogism, which is simply a rule of inference. Rules of inference are merely deductions that guarantee the truth of conclusions drawn from premises if the premises from which they are drawn are true. In the case of the disjunctive syllogism or *modus tollendo ponens*, this rule is:

P or Q;
not P;
therefore, Q.[29]

Self-evidently, this rule also cannot, without more, be used to establish the truth of the premise, 'P or Q,' much less deduce what the unknown cause of the 3-fold difference in MMR was between the two maternity divisions. Nor was Semmelweis able to deduce the cause of childbed fever after excluding all the putative causes, and his inability to elucidate the cause left him dejectedly lamenting, "Everything was uncertain, everything was doubtful, everything was inexplicable, only the enormous number of deaths was an indubitable fact," (SM, 390) as noted in the Introduction.

Semmelweis's account of his discovery

Semmelweis became the Assistant on the first maternity division of the obstetrical department of the AKH on July 1, 1846, his twenty-eighth birthday. He spent a total of 28 months as Assistant in two distinct stints that corresponded to two distinct phases of his discovery: the exclusion of putative causes, and the discovery of the actual cause of childbed fever. The first stint lasted just four months as his predecessor, Franz Breit, was given a two-year extension of his appointment, which required Semmelweis to withdraw as Assistant on October 20, 1846. Semmelweis had planned to spend time in Dublin's Rotunda Hospital, and

[29] Sanford, p. 39.

studied English during the winter of 1846, but changed his plans after Breit was appointed Professor in Tübingen in February 1847. (SM, 391) Before resuming his position as Assistant on March 20, 1847, Semmelweis went to Venice with two friends 'to refresh [his] mind and spirits…among the Venetian art treasures.' (SC, 87). On his return, Semmelweis was shocked to learn of the fateful event that was pivotal in elucidating for him the cause of childbed fever: Kolletschka had died on March 13, 1847.

Exclusion of Putative Causes

By the time Semmelweis became the Assistant, the fact that the MMR from childbed fever on the first maternity division was much higher than on the second had become common knowledge, so much so that patients often begged not to be admitted to the first division (SC, 70). Everyone also knew that since 1941, pursuant to an Imperial Decree issued on October 10, 1840, medical students had been taught only on the first maternity division, and student midwives only on the second maternity division, (SM, 355) yet no one had connected this obvious fact to the differences in the MMR from childbed fever between the two clinics, notwithstanding that several commissions had been convened by the Ministry of Education to investigate the matter. According to Friedrich Wieger, a young doctor who visited Semmelweis from Strasbourg, the measures taken to try to elucidate the cause included frequent changes of bed linen, whitewashing the walls and fumigation of the wards. He also noted that 'the wards of the two services were exchanged. Well! Death followed the first clinic into the ward of the second!' (Wieger, 400)[30]

Semmelweis quickly concluded that 'epidemic influences were not responsible for the horrible devastation of maternity patients in the first clinic,' the term 'epidemic' being a reference not merely to the number of cases but to the causative agent itself: the *genus epidemicus* or atmospheric-cosmic-terrestrial ('telluric') influences. (SC, 64-65) Semmelweis argued that if epidemics caused childbed fever its frequency would not only be the same on the first and second maternity divisions of the AKH, but also the same in the city of Vienna, and, therefore, just as frequent among women who delivered in the street before arriving at the

[30] Kadar & Croft, p.6.

hospital: the so called 'street births.' But it was well known that childbed fever was rare among street births notwithstanding the adverse conditions under which these deliveries occurred. (SC, 81) Moreover, women were admitted to each maternity division on alternate days, except on weekends when they were only admitted to the first division. This clinched the matter for otherwise

> 'one is forced to the unreasonable assumptions that lethal epidemic influences undergo twenty-four-hour remissions and exacerbations and that the remissions, through a series of years, have exactly coincided with admissions to the second clinic, while the exacerbations begin precisely at the time of admission to the first clinic.' (SC, 66)

Semmelweis refuted the commonly held belief that the frequency of childbed fever was seasonal, and more frequent in the winter than summer months, by compiling a table to prove that every month of the year could, in different years, have both the lowest and highest MMR. For example, June was the month with the fewest deaths in 1844, but the month with the greatest number of deaths in 1846. (SM, 360, Table II). Semmelweis also explained with great insight that to the extent that the MMR from childbed fever tended to be higher during the winter months once autopsies became routine, it was because autopsies in the winter months were always performed *before* ward rounds were made on maternity patients at 4PM as it was too dark later in the day to perform autopsies. In the summer months, however, when it was still light after the 4PM ward rounds ended, autopsies tended to be performed *after* the ward rounds as it is was too hot and the smell in the autopsy room too oppressive to perform autopsies earlier in the day. (SM, 444). In other words, women in labour were more likely to be examined after an autopsy in the winter than in the summer. Skoda made no mention whatsoever of these proofs either in his presentation to the College of Professors or in his lecture before the Academy of Sciences on Semmelweis's research (see below). Neither these insights nor their logic owed anything to what Semmelweis had learned from Skoda.

After excluding epidemic causes, and concluding that the cause of the difference in MMR between the two divisions must be endemic,

Semmelweis showed that the difference in MMR could not be explained by any of the many factors to which it had been attributed, such as poor ventilation, laundering of bed linen, diet, the type of patients admitted to the two divisions, because each factor affected both divisions equally or was actually more pronounced in the second division. (SC,75). Particularly ingenious was Semmelweis's proof that overcrowding could not explain the difference in MMR between the two maternity divisions. Overcrowding was widely held to be a contributory cause of childbed fever because epidemics tended to occur in poor, overcrowded cities, but Semmelweis showed that overcrowding was unconnected with deaths from childbed fever.

Since no statistics were kept on overcrowding, Semmelweis used the number of deliveries as a proxy indicator, and determined which month, during the 76 month period, January 1841 to May, 1847 that medical students and midwives had been taught on different divisions, had the greatest number of deliveries and what the MMR from childbed fever was for that month. This was January, 1846, when there were 336 deliveries, and the MMR was 13.4%. Semmelweis then showed that the MMR was greater than 13.4% in 24 of the 76 months, but the number of deliveries were less than 336, i.e. that the MMR was higher when there was less overcrowding. (SM, 364, Table III). Semmelweis also established that there was no temporal correlation between the number of deliveries and MMR by showing that as the number of monthly deliveries declined there was no corresponding decrease in MMR. All which is to say that Semmelweis excluded the putative causes of childbed fever using his native intelligence, not any methodology he learned from Skoda.

After eliminating each putative cause that operated equally on the two dividions, Semmelweis turned his attention to the differences that did exist between the two divisions, and eliminated the existing differences to determine if they had any effect on the MMR from childbed fever. The first difference was the route that the priest took to the 'death chamber' to administer the last rites: the priest could go directly into the death chamber on the second division, but had to pass through five wards to reach the death chamber on the first division, and as he went, an attendant rang a bell that instilled terror into the mothers who heard it. Fear was thought to predispose to childbed fever, so Semmelweis asked the priest to alter his route, which, of course, had no effect on the MMR. (SC, 71, 73) Another existing difference between the two divisions was the position in which women delivered, and so Semmelweis had women deliver in the lateral instead of the dorsal position, as this position was used on the second division, but again, it was, of course, also to no avail. (SC, 87) This was the situation when Semmelweis withdrew as first assistant in October 20, 1846, and caused him to lament about everything being doubtful, questionable, and inexplicable except for the large number of deaths. (SC, 86)

Identifying the cause and spread of childbed fever

By the time Semmelweis was required to withdraw as Assistant on October 20, 1846, he had already made two important observations in the autopsy room relevant to his discovery: first, no newborn had ever died from childbed fever (infection of the newborn) if the mother remained healthy, (SC, 99, 'This explains why an infant never dies of childbed fever while the mother remained healthy'); second, the pathological changes in newborns who died after birth, and who had been born to mothers who died of childbed fever, were the same as those in their mothers, except for the internal genitalia. (SC, 88). After he resumed his position as Assistant on March 20, 1847, learned of Kolletschka's death and reviewed Kolletschka's autopsy report, Semmelweis noted that, except for the internal genitalia, Kolletschka's post-mortem findings were almost identical to the findings he had himself observed at autopsies of women dying of childbed fever, and in their babies. These autopsy findings led Semmelweis to conclude that Kolletschka had died of a disease identical to childbed fever, and that childbed fever was not a disease specific to the puerperium as Rokitansky believed, but a form of pyemia. (SM, 432 'Childbed fever is, accordingly not a species of disease, but a variety of pyemia.')

It is not possible to appreciate the depth of Semmelweis's insights or the logic of his inferences without understanding the two presuppositions on which his reasoning was based. The first was the corollary of a principle Semmelweis learned from Rokitansky: that the pathological changes one observed at autopsy were not 'givens,' but were produced by underlying disease processes.[31] The seed of this concept was sown by the publication of Morgagni's treatise *"On the Seats and Causes of Diseases as investigated by Anatomy,"* in 1761 in Padua, which 'marked the foundation of a new concept of pathology as it developed in the 19th and 20th century.'[32] This new concept was a reaction to the 'philosophes' whose understanding of diseases was derived deductively from theories that were simply conjured up—'a-prioristic postulates,' as Lesky put it (Lesky, 79)—and had no basis in empirical observations. Although '[a]ll the great physicians of the two centuries preceding the publication of Morgagni's work opened the bodies of their deceased patients, anticipating to account for the clinical symptoms as a result of perceptible anatomic changes,' it required Morgagni's 'exceptionally keen mind...to assemble all the pertinent clinical and anatomic facts and to recognize their interrelations.'[33]

By publishing the results of 700 autopsies and the associated case history of each case, and cataloging 'what internal injury is wont to correspond to [what] symptom,'[34] Morgagni 'shifted the emphasis from symptoms to the site of disease,'[35] and firmly established that the symptoms and signs of diseases were merely outward manifestations of abnormalities located in internal organs. Morgagni's English follower, Baillie, extended this idea by noting that 'postmortem appearances are only end-results, although such results may then become again the cause of many symptoms,'[36] which was developed conceptually still further by Bichat and others in Paris 'into the rational science of medicine' whose fundamental aim was to understand 'anatomic lesions as the product of a morbid process.'[37] Rokitansky adopted and developed this principle after he visited Paris with Skoda in 1842, (Lesky, 99), and later wrote in his Handbook of Pathology, 'anatomic alternations of organs and tissues are obviously the result of processes [and] an exact knowledge of these results

---

[31] Klemperer (1961a), p. 377.
[32] Klemperer (1961b), p. 742.
[33] Ibid., p. 743.
[34] Ibid., p. 746.
[35] Porter, 73.
[36] Garrison, p. 355.
[37] Klemperer (1961a), p. 377.

[i.e. the pathologic alterations] was indispensable for acquiring an *insight into the nature of these processes.*'[38] Lesky understood that 'Rokitansky was the first to create a material basis for the concept of "disease process,"' (Lesky, 108), yet failed to see or acknowledge the key role that this concept played in Semmelweis's discovery, and, therefore, her account misses entirely the logic of the deductive inferences that led Semmelweis to his discovery.

Semmelweis reasoned that if the pathological changes observed at autopsy were produced by disease processes, then the same pathological chances must have been produced by the same disease processes. Formally, this conclusion was deductively valid, given the premise, and it is this deduction that was the basis of Semmelweis's striking conclusion that Kolletschka had died of the same disease as mothers who had died of childbed fever:[39]

> 'there was forced on my mind with irresistible clarity…the identity of this disease, of which Kolletschka died, with that from which I had seen so many hundred puerperae die.' (SM391).

The second presupposition on which Semmelweis's inferences depended was that if two diseases are the same, their causes must also be the same. How Semmelweis came by this presupposition is not known, but it is strikingly redolent of the 'rules by which to judge causes and effects' adopted by the Scottish Enlightenment philosopher, David Hume:

> 'where several different objects produce the same effects, it must be by means of some quality, which we discover to be common among them. For as like effects imply like causes, we must always ascribe the causation to the circumstances wherein we discover the resemblance.'[40]

It is, therefore, noteworthy that József Palotay-Purgstaller, a member of the Hungarian Academy of Sciences, who held a doctorate in

---

[38] Ibid. (italics added).
[39] The inference is referred to as modus *ponendo* ponens, not to be confused with the disjuctive syllogism to which Lesky incorrectly imputed Semmelweis's inference, the modus *tollendo* ponens.
[40] Davidson, p. 75.

philosophy and published a philosophical text,[41] taught at the high school (gymnasium) that Semmelweis had attended in Buda (and which became connected to the university after the university moved to Buda in 1777 [and was then moved to Pest in 1783 by Joseph II]); and also that after high school Semmelweis took two classes in philosophy at the University of Pest before entering the University of Vienna in 1839 to study law,[42] which, as noted in the Introduction, likely included courses in logic.

Semmelweis reasoned that if the disease process that killed Kolletschka was the same as the disease process that killed women who died of childbed fever, then the cause of childbed fever must be the same as the cause of the disease process that killed Kolletschka:

> 'The exciting cause of Professor Kolletschka's illness was known… not the wound, but the contamination of the wound by cadaveric particles was the cause of death…[and] if Kolletschka's disease and the disease from which I saw so many puerperae die, are identical, then in the puerperae it must be produced by the self-same engendering cause, which produced it in Kolletschka. In Kolletschka the specific agent was cadaveric particles, which were introduced into the vascular system. I must ask myself the question: Did the cadaveric particles make their way into the vascular systems of the individuals, whom I had seen die of an identical disease? This question I answered in the affirmative.' (SM, 392)[43]

Semmelweis was led to the conclusion that childbed fever was a form of pyemia by the fact that the causative agent was introduced directly into Kolletschka's bloodstream, *yet produced very similar gross pathological changes at autopsy as he found in mothers dying of childbed fever, and in their babies*. He referred to these as 'exudations.' (SM, 429, 'first result of the resorption is disintegration of the blood, and after this the exudates'). The italicized part of Semmelweis's observation informed him that the locations in which he observed pathological changes at autopsy could not have been where the disease started, but were, rather,

[41] Purgstaller.
[42] Antall, p. 121.
[43] Kadar (2020).

the consequences of the disease process (and which also explained why in a few women no pathological abnormalities (exudations) were found at autopsy). (SM, 575-576). And so, ironically, in deducing the cause of childbed fever, Semmelweis was forced to reject his own beloved teacher's theory of childbed fever—which Rokitansky later accepted as correct. (G-Z. 60, see below)—by a chain of inferences that began with the corollary of a principle Semmelweis had learned from Rokitansky himself:

a. If the pathological findings are the same, they must have been produced by the same underlying disease process, and be the same disease, (SM, 558, 'since the findings on cadavers dead from pyemia are identical with those dead of childbed fever, then childbed fever is the same disease');

b. If the diseases are the same, their causes must be the same, (SM, 558, 'if it is the same disease, then it must have the same cause');

c. The underlying cause of Kolletschka's death was the introduction of cadaveric particles into his blood stream by a cut to his finger;

d. Therefore, the cause of childbed fever must be the introduction of cadaveric particles introduced into the blood stream of mothers in labor.

Semmelweis had by then realized that babies contracted the infection via the blood stream—i.e. from their mother's blood through the placenta and not after birth—from the fact that babies never died of infection if their mothers had not died of childbed fever. (SM, 402). Semmelweis concluded that the causative agent could similarly gain access to the blood stream of mothers dying of childbed fever through the raw surface of the placental bed—where the placenta had been attached to the uterus during pregnancy:

> 'In gravidae, parturients or puerperae, there is a place in the body, which has no epidermis or epithelium, and that is the internal surface of the uterus; starting from the internal os

> upwards, this is the absorption place for the decomposed matter which causes puerperal fever. If wounds are caused by labour, then every place on the genitals, indeed any wound on the body, can be the site of absorption.' (SM, 504).

It was only at this juncture in the sequence of observations—i.e. after Kolletschka's death linked deaths from childbed fever to autopsies—that the characteristic odor on the hands of medical students and attendants engaged in autopsies—which could linger for long periods after they washed their hands with soap and water—entered into the chain of inferences of how mothers contracted the infection:

> 'That the cadaveric particles clinging to the hands are not entirely removed by the ordinary method of washing the hands with soap and water, is shown by the cadaveric odour, which the hands retain for a longer or shorter time. During the examination of gravidae, parturients, and puerperae, the hand contaminated with cadaveric particles is brought into contact with the genitals of these individuals, and hence the possibility of absorption, and by means of absorption, introduction of cadaveric particles into the vascular system of these individuals is postulated, and by this means the same disease is produced in these puerperae, which we saw in Kolletschka.' (SM, 392).

And it was only after Semmelweis had concluded the cadaveric particles could be the cause of childbed fever that he deduced the cause of the difference in MMR between the two divisions:

> '*After it became evident* that the preponderance of mortality in the First Clinic in contrast with the Second was to be sought in the cadaveric and ichorous particles, with which the hands of the examiners were contaminated, *the previously inexplicable phenomena*, which took place in the First Division, *could be very easily explained.*' (SM, 401, italics added).

In other words, it was only after Semmelweis had deduced the cause of childbed fever and how it was transmitted that he realized that the disproportionately high MMR on the first division could be explained by the fact that midwives were taught only on the second division, and were not engaged in autopsies—but the fact that student midwives and medical students were taught on different divisions of the lying-in hospital played no role in the inferences that led to Semmelweis theory of causation in the first place, contrary to the account Skoda gave to the Academy of Sciences on October 18, 1849 of Semmelweis's discovery (see below). Of all the philosophers of science who have written about Semmelweis's reasoning, Alexader Bird has been the only one to understand the correct sequence of his inferences:

> 'The significance of Kolletschka's death is that it drew Semmelweis's attention to a difference between the midwives and the students that might otherwise have gone unnoticed—the fact that they attended autopsies and carried out dissections before performing examinations in the wards.'[44]

And the difference *had* gone unnoticed by several commissions appointed by the Ministry of Education to look into the high MMR on the first maternity clinic. [**M, 24**].

So it can be seen that Lesky's account of Semmelweis discovery turned the sequence of inferences on its head. According to Lesky, once all the putative causes of childbed fever had been excluded Semmelweis was able to deduce the cause of childbed fever from the fact that medical students and midwives were taught on different divisions and only medical students were involved in autopsies, plus odor that lingered on the hands of those involved in autopsies. But there is historical evidence refuting this sequence of events independent of Semmelweis's own subsequent account.

A commission, conducting an investigation just after Semmelweis was required to withdraw as the Assistant, concluded that the difference in MMR between the two clinics was caused by trauma to the birth canal of mothers inflicted by rough examinations performed by the many foreign medical students who were taught on the first division, and, as a consequence, their number was reduced from 40 to 20 at the end of 1846, after which the MMR from childbed fever did decrease somewhat. [**M, 24**] In other words, the putative cause—rough examinations by foreign medical students—took into consideration that medical students and

[44] Bird, p. 348.

midwives were taught on different divisions, but this did not lead to a correct conclusion about the cause. Semmelweis dismissed the explanation as absurd, pointing out that the baby's passage through the birth canal was so much more traumatic that if rough examinations could cause childbed fever, one had to wonder why every delivery did not end fatally:

> 'The cause of the greater mortality in the First Obstetrical Clinic has been attributed to the fact that the accoucheurs examined more roughly than do pupil-midwives. Granted that it be so, if the… rough introduction of the index-finger into the vagina widened and lengthened by pregnancy… be such a harmful thing that it may cause such a fearful condition as puerperal fever is, then indeed passage of the fetal body through the genitals must be just as harmful, so that it cannot be imagined why each birth does not end fatally.' (SM, 377)

Lesky's rejection of Semmelweis's account

Lesky rejected Semmelweis's account, and the pivotal role that Kolletschka's death played in his discovery, *tout court*. She accepted instead Podach's argument that Semmelweis's account must have been an after-the-fact reconstruction:

> 'As for the pathological-anatomical premise of Semmelweis's discovery, this was placed in a correct light by E. F. Podach's profound and advanced work on the structure of puerperal anatomy of the time. Although he has deprived Semmelweis's discovery of its romantic aura of a lightning accidental discovery in connection with the Kolletschka case, *it made visible for the first time the hard pathologic-anatomical work that Semmelweis had actually done*. Podach showed that it required years of training and experience in systematic pathologic-anatomical thinking until Semmelweis was able to override the view of his teacher Rokitansky of the supposed specificity of puerperal pyaemia, and to view the anatomical changes in the corpses of mothers and their newborns, as well as those in Kolletschka's corpse, as those of pyemia.' [**M-56, 57**]

Exactly so, only Podach concluded that Semmelweis could not have had the requisite experience in anatomic pathology to make these connections and inferences, and even speculated that Semmelweis's delay in publishing his research may have reflected a subconscious desire to avoid having to contradict his teacher, Rokitansky:

> 'The 'Kolletschka case' was not only emphasized by an agitated mind, but also by a probably semi-conscious, half unconscious purpose. It made it possible for Semmelweis to avoid the unpleasant task of dealing expressly with his discredited teacher in public, and thus to explicitly refute Rokitansky's ideas about childbed fever. That it would have required a systematic statement may be why Semmelweis had so long opposed to the detailed publication of his discovery.' (P, 873).

Why Lesky accepted Podach's argument, given that she knew its premise was untrue, is open to question. What is clear, however, is that Lesky knew the extent of Semmelweis's autopsy experience because, as previously noted, she acknowledged in her book about the Vienna Medical School that '[t]he fact that in 1844 Rokitansky made available to him all female cadavers at the pathological institute was undoubtedly of great importance to Semmelweis,' (Lesky, 185), and in her monograph went even further, and acknowledged that by also examining and dissecting female cadavers who had died of gynaecological diseases, Semmelweis became 'a pioneer of gynecological diagnoses in Vienna,' and the teacher of his former teachers, Chiari and Arneth, in gynecology. [**M-92**].

Podach supported his conclusion by the fact that neither Hebra, Routh, Haller, nor Skoda mentioned Kolletschka's death in their reports of Semmelweis's discovery, nor was Kolletschka's death mentioned in the minutes of the meeting of the Imperial Society of Physician at which Semmelweis first presented his discovery on May 15, 1850. (P, 873) However, none of these reports were primarily concerned with *how* the discovery was made, but with what the discovery was, and with the effectiveness of prophylactic chlorine hand-disinfection. Indeed, the specific intent of each publication, except Skoda's, was to persuade their audiences to adopt Semmelweis's prophylaxis.

Negative historical evidence is weak evidence that something did not occur. For example, Hebra, Haller, and Skoda also did not mention that Semmelweis's prophylaxis included scrubbing the fingernails with a nail brush, but that does not mean a nail brush was not used: Wieger, an eyewitness to how chlorine hand-disinfection was practiced, characterized it as the whole secret of the disinfection. (Wieger, 400)[45] Moreover, the following statement in the minutes of Semmelweis's lecture to the Society of Physicians on May 15, 1850 may fairly be construed as a reference to how Kolletschka's death led Semmelweis to his discovery without mentioning Kolletschka by name:

> 'the pathological-anatomical findings in childbed fever, *which bears the greatest resemblance to pyaemia in anatomists and surgeons after wounding and impregnating their freshly injured bodies with rotten organic matter from corpses,* led Dr. Semmelweis to the conviction that puerperal fever is likewise a pyemic process produced by the absorption of rotting organic matter from the inner lining of the uterus into the blood of the mother…' (vGy, 49, Appendix C, p. 177-178, italics added)

Benedek has also cited hearsay evidence by the Hungarian, Ödön Tuszkai, who visited London in 1908 to speak with the elderly Routh—who as a young doctor had visited Semmelweis from England in 1847—and noted that Routh had told Tuszkai that he (Routh) had heard 'directly from Semmelweis's own mouth' how tremendously excited Semmelweis was by the coincidence that Kolletschka's autopsy findings were the same as those of mothers dying of childbed fever. (B, 89-90) But the most direct affirmative evidence that Kolletschka's death did indeed provide the vital clue that led to Semmelweis's theory, comes from Kussmaul's memoirs in which Kussmaul wrote the following concerning Semmelweis and Kolletschka:

> 'Of all the acquaintances I made in Vienna, my memory of Semmelweis is the most pleasant and appreciated. We first came to know him *shortly before* he had made the great beneficial discovery which mankind owes to him; it occupied him continually and was the subject of our daily conversations with this excellent man….The light unexpectedly came to him on the occasion of the autopsy of a highly esteemed colleague, the professor of anatomy, Kolletschka, that finally elucidated

45 Kadar & Croft, p.3.

for him the true nature and cause of the murderous disease he had so longed for.

Kolletschka had contracted poison from a corpse through an injured finger, and succumbed to it on March 13, 1847. Semmelweis attended the funeral. His findings surprised him immensely, and agreed with his findings in those who had died of childbed fever. That could not be a coincidence. He concluded that the same foul poison that killed the anatomist also killed the women who were giving birth. In the case of Kolletschka, the blood was penetrated through the injured finger, while in the case of women who gave birth, it was penetrated through the parts of the body injured during birth. The anatomist had himself put the poison into his own body, and the women who had given birth came by it through fingers that had come into contact with rotting substances.—A previously striking, unexplained fact found its simple explanation.' (K, 173-174, italics added)

Although Kussmaul wrote his autobiography in 1899, three years before his death, it was based on his own personal remembrances. Kussmaul was not an obstetrician, and had no axe to grind; moreover, Kussmaul said he arrived in Vienna *before* Semmelweis made his discovery, and was in a position to know first-hand what role Kolletschka's death played in that discovery. Lesky must have been aware of what Kussmaul had written for she cited to Kussmaul's autobiography for a different proposition in a footnote in her monograph, [**M, 57**, n. 116], yet made no mention of what Kussmaul had written concerning the relationship between Kolletschka's death and Semmelweis's conclusions about the cause of childbed fever.

Semmelweis's chlorine hand-disinfection experiment

Semmelweis's shrewd inferences only netted him a theory, which he now had to prove, and there were several ways in which he could have proved that medical students and attendants were transporting the infective material from the autopsy room to the labor ward. (SM, 578). The method Semmelweis chose was to remove the cause and see if this prevented the disease; it was a based on a principle that Vonka and Gillies have shown dates back to at least the 13th century, and was expressed by Thomas Aquinas (1225-1274) in the maxim *sublata causa, tolitur effectus* ("if the cause is removed, the effect is taken away").[46] Although Vonca and Gillies gave priority to Claude Bernard, who cited the maxim in his *Introduction to the Study of Experimental Medicine*, publication in 1865, the year Semmelweis died, Semmelweis clearly applied Aquinas's maxim before Bernard, even if he did not cite the maxim, implying that he was not aware of it. To understand Semmelweis's reasoning, and the rationale of the animal experiments he later conducted, it is necessary to understand the causal ideas that animated Semmelweis's actions, but no biographer besides Carter has given any thought to this fundamental aspect of Semmelweis's reasoning.[47]

Causation, the idea that one thing or event brings about another thing or event, has been conceptualized in a number of different ways, one of the commonest being in terms of necessary and sufficient causes.[48] C is said to be a *sufficient* cause E, if whenever the cause, C, occurs its effect, E, occurs (expressed as 'if C, then E'); C is said to be a *necessary* cause of E, if whenever the event, E, occurs, its cause, C, also occurs (expressed as 'if E, then C,' or, equivalently, 'E only if C'). It follows from the definition of necessary causation that by removing a necessary cause one can prevent the disease; and this is expresses by the deductively valid inference referred to as *modus tollendo tollens*;

If D, then C:
not-C,
therefore, not-D.

Although Semmelweis did not use this terminology, he clearly understood the logical difference between a sufficient and a necessary cause.[49]

Semmelweis defined the cause of childbed fever in terms of its necessary, *sine qua non*, cause. (SM, 505). Carter has shown that Semmelweis was the first to define a disease in terms of its cause, and that

---

46 Vonka, p. 1835; Gillies (2019), p. 29, n. 3.
47 Kadar (2020).
48 Sosa & Tooley, pp. 5-8.
49 Kadar (2020).

by doing so likely influenced the development of germ theory[50] and modern concepts of disease.[51] Semmelweis's definition of childbed fever in terms of a necessary cause was not accidental: Semmelweis expressly rejected defining the disease in terms of a sufficient cause, even if, as noted, he did not use the necessary-sufficient terminology.

Hamernik, an internist from Prague, (Lesky, 121, 187), rejected Semmelweis's proof of causation, and contended that for any 'factor to be considered as a cause of an existent disease…the following questions must be answered in the affirmative every time:'

> 1. Has this cause always the same result?
> 2. Can the disease under consideration be produced experimentally every time in this manner?
> 3. In those cases where the disease is not caused by this factor, can the actual cause of the abortive experiment be assigned? (SM, 672).

These are, as Carter has pointed out, all criteria of causal sufficiency, (SC, 37), and Semmelweis expressly rejected them, saying that the 'true cause' (aetiology) of a disease is its necessary, *sine qua non*, cause, (SC, 149). In his reply to Hamernik, Semmewleis expressly distinguished his own (necessary) cause as being different from Hamernik's (sufficient) cause, but stressed that his animal experiments (see below) had established that what he had identified as the necessary cause of childbed fever—decaying animal organic matter—could also be a sufficient cause of pyemia and induce pathological changes in animals indistinguishable from those found at autopsy in women dying of childbed fever, i.e. could be both a necessary cause, and, contingently, a sufficient cause—contingent on there being a site of ingress into the blood stream (see below), and on the decaying animal-organic matter having reached a sufficient degree of putrefaction (SM, 575-576). His response to Hamernik was:

---

[50] Carter (1985).
[51] Carter (2003).

> The first condition is unfounded. The reader knows that I have injected rabbits with decaying matter; some consequently died of pyemia and others did not. Could we deny that the decaying matter was the cause of the pyemia in the rabbits that died simply because the matter did not occasion pyemia in all the rabbits? I have fulfilled the second condition: I have produced puerperal fever experimentally in rabbits in this way. I have not fulfilled the third condition: I cannot explain why a few rabbits did not develop pyemia. However, instead, *my aetiology of childbed fever satisfies another condition* that Hammernik had not posed but one that constitutes a condition for a true aetiology. Namely, I have reduced the disease by making harmless that which I have identified as its cause. (SC, 216, italics added).

Semmelweis chose to prove his theory that decaying animal-organic matter was a necessary cause of childbed fever by proving that removal of what he contended was the necessary cause would prevent the disease:

> 'If the hypothesis is correct, that the hand-borne cadaveric particles produce the same disease in puerperae, which the cadaveric particles clinging to the knife caused in Kolletschka, then, if by a chemical effect they may be completely destroyed on the hand…this disease can be prevented *to the extent that it is dependent upon the effect of cadaveric particles carried by the examining finger*.' (SM, 393)

In other words, Semmelweis's reasoning was based on the *modus tollendo tollens* and not, as Lesky claimed, on the *modus tollendo ponens* inference; nor did his rationale have anything to do with the 'statistical methods' that Lesky claimed Semmelweis 'learned to handle' from Skoda. **[M, 60]**

Using the characteristic odor on the attendants' hands as the end-point, Semmelweis determined that this could be done by disinfecting the hands with a chlorine solution and carefully scrubbing 'the nails and the skin folds surrounding the nails with the most scrupulous care.' (Wieger, 401)[52] With the permission of his chief, Johann Klein, Semmelweis

[52] Kadar & Croft, p.6.

implemented hand-disinfection at the end of May, 1847, and after it successfully reduced the MMR from childbed fever, he concluded that his theory was correct:

> I have assumed that the cadaveric material adhering to the examining hand of the accoucheur is the cause of the greater mortality in the First Obstetrical Clinic; I have eliminated this factor by the introduction of the chlorine washings… The conclusion, therefore, that the cadaveric particles adhering to the hand had in reality caused the preponderant mortality in the Frist Clinic, was also a correct one. (SM, 395)

But there was a glitch. The MMR on the first division fell immediately after the chlorine disinfection was started, and remained low for three months— falling to 2.4%, 1.2% and 1.9%, in June, July, August, 1847, respectively—but then spiked again in September, October, November to 5.2%, 4%, and 5%, respectively. Semmelweis quickly realized that the increase in September was caused by negligent hand-disinfection by some of the new intake of medical students (who were identified by having the names of the medical student and midwife assigned to each mother recorded in the mother's medical records), (Wieger, 400)[53], but the causes of the increase in October and November were very different, and enabled Semmelweis to refine his theory both as to the source of the causative agent, and the means by which it could reach the genital tract of mothers.[54]

In October, a mother with carcinoma of the uterus was admitted to the bed in the maternity ward where ward rounds always started, and was followed by an outbreak of childbed fever in 11 of 12 mothers serially, 'in a row' on the ward. (SM, 392). The reason was that when Semmelweis first implemented chlorine hand-disinfection he only required attendants to disinfect their hands before entering the labour ward, but once on the ward, they were permitted to wash their hands between examining patients with soap and water, as he believed that once on the ward the attendants' hands 'could not become contaminated again.' (SC, 93) So the causative agent was spread from the mother with the infected carcinoma of the

[53] Kadar & Croft. (see supplemental material)
[54] Kadar 2020.

uterus successively to others mothers by their examiners. This episode made Semmelweis realize that decomposing animal organic matter could also come from 'ichorous [purulent] discharges' of living persons as well as cadavers, and that hand-disinfection was required before any mother was examined in labour to prevent childbed fever.

In November, 1847, a pregnant woman was admitted who had a 'discharging carious left knee,' but normal genitalia. By that time, chlorine hand-disinfection prior to every examination had been implemented; nevertheless, eleven mothers in the same room as this patient succumbed to childbed fever. Semmelweis could tell by the odor that 'ichorous exhalations [discharge] of the carious knee completely saturated the air of her ward,' and concluded that *in these limited cases*—not *tout court* as under the miasmatic theory of epidemics, and as the historian, David Wootton, incorrectly believed[55]— the cause of childbed fever could be construed as a miasma, and that such patients needed to be isolated:

> 'If in a ward there are one or more sick pueperae among the healthy ones, and if their disease, whether puerperal fever or *other disease*, gives off decomposed matter, then this exhaled decomposed matter will cause childbed fever if it penetrates into the genital organs of the healthy puerperae along with the atmospheric air of the lying-in room. If the foregoing is understood as "puerperal miasma" then I agree. Anything beyond that does not exist as puerperal miasma…Thereafter, such individuals were isolated to prevent similar tragedies.' (SM, 542-543, italics added).

Thus, Semmelweis quickly assimilated the new evidence he was confronted with to deepen his understanding of how the disease was caused and spread, and how it could be prevented. The necessary ('sine qua non') cause was decaying animal-organic matter whose source could be 'a diseased person of any age, sex, regardless of whether the person suffers from childbed fever,' which was transferred to the mother by 'examining fingers, operating hands, instruments…[or] anything that is contaminated by animal-organic matter,' and then resorbed through

---

[55] Wootton, p. 222.

damaged skin or mucous membranes or 'any point of the body that is stripped of epidermis and epithelium.' (SM, 430).

Skoda's account of Semmelweis's discovery

The account Skoda gave of Semmelweis's discovery before the Academy of Sciences completely severed Semmelweis's discovery from its anatomic-pathological foundations. Skoda began his account by describing the view of the 'Viennese School of Anatomic Pathology' of the pathogenesis of childbed fever, according to which the disease began most commonly with:

> 'exudation at the wound on the inner surface of the uterus at the placental insertion site; or—less commonly—with partial or total conversion of the contents of a single or all the veins of the uterus to pus, with previous or subsequent exudation from the vein walls; or, finally, with an exudation on the peritoneum.' (vGy, 38; Appendix A, p.164)

Skoda then presented what Semmelweis had discovered—that childbed fever was a form of pyemia caused by decaying animal-organic matter—as something that was already known:

> 'Pyemia without suppuration or analogous suppurative changes in the organs arises from the action of rotting animal substance on the blood.' (vGy 39; Appendix A, p.165)

In cases of childbed fever the source of this material could not be 'the putrefaction that develops in uterine or vaginal secretions under ordinary influences or the peculiar nature of the fluids of recently delivered women because this could not account for the often mentioned unequal number of sickenings in the two departments,' and, according to Skoda, this led Semmelweis to conclude that the rotting substances must come from outside, and that the source of the material had to be the morgue:

> 'After Dr. Semmelweis . . . considered all the circumstances for a few months, he realized that both he and the students frequently examined corpses, that the cadaverous odor on their hands disappears only after a long time, despite washing several times, and that he and the students often crossed directly from *examining cadavers to the examination of the woman giving*

> *birth, was the only possible way of transferring a putrid animal substance to the birth site of the mothers.* This was at the same time *only one among the possible causes of puerperal disease*, which on the distribution for midwives was either not at all effective or extremely limited, so that, assuming this cause, the very unequal number of diseases in the two departments would be very understandable.' (vGy, 39; Appendix A, p165, italics added)

In other words, Skoda told the Academy that Semmelweis realized that the rotting animal matter that causes pyemia could not be a specific product of puerperal women as this could not explain the difference in MMR between the two divisions. And it was this fact, Skoda claimed, that led Semmelweis to conclude that 'rotting animal matter' must come from outside, and after excluding other factors, concluded, from the smell that lingered on the hands of medical students and attendants engaged in autopsies long after they washed their hands with soap and water, that the rotting matter must have been transported from the autopsy room to the labor ward. This was not how Semmelweis deduced the cause of childbed fever, and it was not a correct account of his theory. Moreover, Skoda knew that cadavers were not the only source of the causative agent as Hebra had reported that the causative agent could come from living persons in December, 1847, almost two years earlier. But it was a very plausible account; indeed it was so plausible that it caused Podach to conclude:

> 'Not Semmelweis, but J. Skoda, not the work of Semmelweis from the year 1861, but the Academy lecture of Skoda from the year 1849, is the authoritative source for the origin and foundation of the doctrine of child bed fever.' (P, 873)

Only the justification Podach gave for accepting Skoda's account over Semmelweis's own account of his discovery is not something the available historical evidence supports, much less compels us to believe, and what Skoda described was not only an incorrect account of how Semmelweis was led to his discovery, it was also not an accurate account of Semmelweis's theory. Far from concluding that infection could not originate from the mother's own genital tract, Semmelweis concluded that decaying organic matter *could* indeed be generated within the mother's own birth canal, and cause what Semmelweis called 'autoinfection':

> 'As for the etiological factors which cause the formation of a decomposed matter within the individual and thereby causes childbed fever through auto-infection, they are the following:
>
> Decomposition of the normal lochial flow, as a result of a rather prolonged retention of the lochial discharge from whatever cause, retention of blood clots in the uterine cavity after haemorrhage, retention of the placenta or placental and membranous remnants, bruising of the genital organs as a result of a prolonged stage of expulsion, or as a result of necrosing perineal lacerations after operations.' (SM 552).

These cases could obviously not be prevented by chlorine hand-disinfection because they originated from within the mothers' own genital tracts. However, Semmelweis did describe the measures that needed to be taken to minimize these infections: avoid prolonged second stage labors, and pendular rotations of the forceps to effect delivery; remove any placental remnants and blood to prevent their absorption into the blood stream. (SM, 557).

It is true, as Skoda told the Academy, that it was known that 'wounds acquired during autopsies can results in pyemia,' (SM, 558), but what was not known is that childbed fever was a form of pyemia or could be caused in the same way. This is what Semmelweis discovered by noting that the pathological changes that follow 'wounds acquired during autopsies'—i.e. the post-mortem findings in Kolletschka—were identical to the pathological changes found in women dying from childbed fever, with the exception of the internal genitalia. Indeed, Lesky acknowledge that Semmelweis had arrived at a 'new version of the term puerperal fever in this synopsis of pathological-anatomy that went beyond Rokitansky.' [**M-57**] And that is why after excluding all the putative causes Semmelweis was unable to deduce the cause of the difference in MMR between the two maternity divisions. Skoda was correct that Semmelweis based his theory of how 'rotting or decaying substances' reached 'the mother's womb' on the odor on the hands of the attendants involved in autopsy, but this was only *after* Semmelweis realized that the causative agent— the 'rotting or decaying substances,' as Skoda put it— came from cadavers (and soon thereafter realized that it could also come from living persons). This was not known; it is what Semmelweis discovered; and this is why several commissions had not been able to deduce the cause of the high MMR on the first maternity division before Semmelweis discovered the cause. And it was likely this account by Skoda that caused Semmelweis to make the already quoted comment at the end of his response to Scanzoni's criticism of the animal experiments Skoda had described in his lecture:

> 'Scanzoni...has not even been able to learn the true cause of childbed fever from Skoda's discourse, who had indeed mentioned some things not pertaining to puerperal fever.' (SC, 173-174)

Why Semmelweis conducted animal experiments with Lautner

'To ask why an event happened is to ask, in some sense, for a causal explanation of the event.'[56] However, two very different concepts of causation are implicated in the question of why Semmelweis conducted the Lautner experiments that apply to two very different types of subject matter.

Causal concepts of sufficiency and necessity apply to the subject matter of natural science, such as the cause of childbed fever, as already discussed, but very different notions of causation apply to the subject matter of history, which mostly consists of the actions of human beings, such as Semmelweis's decision to conduct animal experiments, to delay publishing his results, to leave Vienna in October, 1850.[57] Why Semmelweis conducted the Lautner experiments implicates both types of causation. Therefore, it is a two-part question that requires a two-part answer: (1) what induced or motivated Semmelweis to conduct these experiments in the first place, and (2) what was their intended purpose, i.e.

---

[56] Debbins, p. xxii.

[57] Collingood (1993), pp. 213-217.

what was Semmelweis trying to demonstrate or prove with these experiments?[58]

What motivated Semmelweis to conduct the Lautner experiments implicates concepts of agency, which were, historically, the earliest conceptualization of causation. Under agency concepts, what is 'caused' is 'the free and deliberate act of a conscious and responsible agent:' here, the Lautner experiments. What causes the act, referred to as the *causa quod* or efficient cause of the act, 'is a situation or state of things existing,' and known by the agent to be existing; it is the agent's motivation for acting. The agent's purpose in acting, referred to as the *causa ut* or final cause of the act, is 'the state of things to be brought about.' Neither a *causa quod* nor a *causa ut* could be a cause if the other were absent.[59]

The 'situation or state of things existing' that motivated Semmelweis to conduct animal experiments with Lautner—the *causa quod* of the Lautner experiments—was that Klein did not accept that the results of the chlorine hand-disinfection experiment proved Semmelweis's theory. Just because the MMR from childbed fever fell after chlorine hand-disinfection was implemented, it did not mean that the chlorine hand-disinfection had caused the MMR to fall: *post hoc* did not mean *propter hoc*. Klein simply attributed the fall in MMR to the fact that the chlorine hand-disinfection was implemented after the epidemic causing the childbed fever had abated—and the very documents Lesky discovered brought this information to light. Klein noted in his objection the Skoda's motion to the College of Professors:

> '*After the epidemic of childbed fever ceased in the year 1847, the undersigned introduced chlorine washings on his clinic* on the recommendation of his assistant... But the matter—as Professor Skoda has himself agreed—remained unclear, and had by no means been decided...'[**M, 29,** italics added]

Klein repeated the same objection in his letter to the Ministry of Education explaining why he had denied Semmelweis's request for an extension of his Assistantship:

---

[58] Kadar (2020).
[59] Collingwood (2014), p. 292.

> 'It is by no means clear from the fact that since the termination of the last epidemic of childbed fever the mortality rate is lower, *that it is the result of chlorine washes*, that the cause of the childbed epidemic has been found, and its recurrence was prevented. For this the experiment is still too young, and therefore the appropriation of so much merit by Semmelweis is still premature and presumptuous.' [**M, 46** §(e), italics added].

Klein's objection was shared by others both inside and outside Vienna. For example, Eduard Lumpe, who had been Assistant on the first maternity division during 1940-1942, (Lesky, 182), also based his objection on the wide fluctuations in the frequency of childbed fever. He argued that during the time he was the Assistant, 'there was such a difference between the maximum and minimum mortality that one could think of nearly everything else but a common invariable cause.' (SM, 694).

The Editors of the *Gazette Médicale de Paris* raised similar objections to the chlorine hand-disinfection experiment. Wieger, who visited Semmelweis in 1847, and remained in contact with Semmelweis, published an article in the *Gazette Médicale de Strasbourg* on April 20, 1849 that presented for the first time the annual MMR from childbed fever on the first maternity division of the AKH for the years 1841-1848, inclusive; he also described how chlorine hand-disinfection was actually practiced, (Wieger, 401),[60] and added a case report that confirmed Semmelweis's observation that decomposing animal-organic matter could come from living persons, (Wieger, 402).[61] The article engendered the following editorial comments:

> 'We do not wish to assert that the doctrine derived from these facts is intrinsically and completely erroneous; we simply believe that this doctrine does not follow logically from these facts; for example, the remarkable fall *over a year and a half*, starting from when the hand washing measure was put into practice, could be due to a completely different circumstance. Who is not familiar with the capricious and singular

[60] Kadar & Croft, p.3.
[61] Ibid.

> fluctuations of epidemics, and especially of epidemics of puerperal fever?' (Ed, 383, italics in original)[62]

The same concern was also later expressed with specific reference to Semmelweis's results by Joseph Hermann Schmidt, Professor of Obstetrics in Berlin, in a letter dated August, 28 1850, to Brücke, who had informed Schmidt of Semmelweis's work. Semmelweis quoted the following from the letter in an article published in 1858 in which Semmelweis first described his work:

> 'I regard the surprising observation of S. [Semmelweis] the more worthy of interest because you [Brücke] confirm it yourself, for you are not only a physiologist, but are also, with regard to the *post hoc ergo propter hoc*, more sceptical than credulous.' (vGy, 69, italics added).

In other words, Schmidt was prepared to accept Semmelweis's observations only because they had been confirmed by Brücke, and because Brücke himself was more skeptical than credulous of before and after experimental proofs.

But the most unequivocal evidence that there was widely held concern among physicians at that time about the fallacy of this line of reasoning from before-and-after (diachronic) clinical experiments is provided by the letter Semmelweis received from a Dr. Everken, Director of the Royal Midwives Institute in Paderborn, Germany in 1858, to whom Semmelweis had written to ask if Everken had used chlorine hand-disinfection, and if so, what effect it had had. After recounting his experience with chlorine hand-disinfection, Everken concluded his letter with:

> 'You will concede, most honored colleague, that it is difficult to make a decision and that the conclusion *post hoc, ergo proper hoc* is perhaps nowhere more deceptive than in medicine.' (SM, 712).

Evidence that Semmelweis and the young doctors visiting him understood this criticism only came to light after Lesky's death with the

---

[62] Kadar & Croft, p. 3.

discovery of the letter that another young doctor visiting Semmelweis, Heinrich Hermann Schwartz, wrote to his professor in Kiel, Gustav Adolf Michaelis, to report on Semmelweis's theory and the results of the chlorine hand-disinfection experiment:

> 'Therefore, the washing of hands with dilute sulfuric acid or *chlorine liquida* was required of all the hospital practitioners after involvement with corpses and before examination of those giving birth. And while one dare not with certainty declare *propter hoc*, one can at least say *post hoc*, given the remarkable change that has occurred in the sanitary conditions of the institution (italics in original translation).'[63]

This letter was dated of December 21, 1847, and, therefore, was written before any objections or criticisms of Semmelweis's proof could have been received from outside the AKH for Semmelweis's discovery was only communicated to the medical community in the same month, December, 1847, by Hebra's Editorial. (SM, 566-567). Semmelweis never saw Schwarz's letter, (SM, 575), and, therefore, it could be argued that this objection may have concerned Schwarz but not necessarily Semmelweis. However, this seems unlikely given that Semmelweis discussed his theory with the young doctors visiting him daily, a detail Kussmaul recorded in his memoirs, writing that Semmelweis's 'great, beneficial discovery…occupied him constantly, and was the subject of our daily conversations with this excellent man.' (K, 173).

So Semmelweis conducted animal experiments to counter this objection to the results of the chlorine hand-disinfection experiment, but what specifically was he trying to achieve that would counter this objection? Semmelweis first response was to provide corroborating statistical evidence that the high rates of childbed fever on the first maternity division were tied to autopsies. He did this by showing that the MMR from childbed fever first increased sharply at the AKH after 1823, when autopsies first started to be performed routinely at the hospital. There was only one maternity division at that time, but Semmelweis also showed that after the second maternity division was created in 1833 (because

[63] Carter & Tate, p. 256.

additional building had been added to the hospital, including 600 maternity beds) the MMR from childbed fever remained the same on the two maternity divisions until 1941, and only became persistently higher on the first maternity division after medical students and pupil midwives were taught on separate divisions pursuant to an order from the Ministry of Education. (SM, 397-399)

Presumably this was the 'crowning statistical proof' that Lesky was referring to as the third prong of Semmelweis's discovery (see above), but this evidence, like the evidence from the chlorine hand-disinfection experiment, was indirect. The chlorine hand-disinfection experiment had proved that 'decaying animal organic matter' was a necessary cause of childbed fever, and the statistical evidence proved an association between childbed fever and autopsies. But to meet the objections that his proof relied on the *post hoc ergo propter hoc* fallacy, Semmelweis wanted to prove that what he postulated was the cause could actually bring about the disease. He expressed this by saying that he wanted to prove his theory "directly," and that is why he conducted animal experiments. (SM 408—'In order to submit my theory to a direct test, I considered that animal experiments were necessary). Specifically, Semmelweis wanted to prove that not only could he prevent the disease by removing its putative cause, but he could also induce the same disease process as childbed fever in animals by proving that material from cadavers could induce the same pathological changes in animals as is observed in mothers dying of childbed fever. In other words, he wanted to prove that decaying animal-organic could also be a *sufficient* cause.

Semmelweis likely planned to conduct animal experiments with Lautner towards the end of 1848, after he felt he had sufficient follow-up to prove that chlorine hand-disinfection was effective, but was prevented from doing so by Lautner's arrest following the October riots. [**M, 80**] This seems the most reasonable interpretation of the fact that in his *Lehre* Semmelweis inverted the chronology of the Lautner experiments and his application for an extension of his assistantship, and wrote the following about the Lautner experiments:

> 'In order to submit my theory to a direct test, I considered that animal experiments were necessary, which I performed on

> rabbits along with my friend, Dr. Lautner, assistant to Professor Rokitansky.' (SM, 409)

After describing each of the nine experiments, Semmelweis wrote:

> 'As the end of my two-year service drew near, I requested that my period of service be increased two years also, as had been done for my predecessor, Dr. Breit, and of course, I thought that I was bound even more to request it, as I would thus have the opportunity to be able to confirm my views on the origin of childbed fever, which raised so many contradictions, by a study of two years longer, but my petition was in vain even though this was given to my colleagues serving in the second division.' (SM, 412)

This implied a chronology that was the inverse of the actual chronology, and the most likely explanation for it is that, writing eleven years after the fact, Semmelweis conflated when he planned to conduct the experiments with when he actually conducted them. In keeping with this is that Semmelweis often recounted autobiographical details rather casually, paying little heed to factual details. For example, Semmelweis gave the following, equally misleading account of his application for a docent on February 9, 1850, for which Lesky took him to task:

> 'After my retirement, on March 20, 1849, from the post of Assistant,
>
> I requested a Privat-Docent in Midwifery. My petition was without success.' (SM, 412)

Semmelweis conducted nine experiments in domestic rabbits with Lautner, and described each experiment in detail in his *Lehre*, (SM, 409-412), as did Skoda in his lecture to the Academy of Sciences. (cGy, 42-45; Appendix A, p168-172) The first experiment was started on March 22, 1849, three days after Semmelweis's Assistantship ended; the last was begun on August 8, 1849, and ended with the animal's death on August 20. Each experiment consisted of introducing blood and other fluids from corpses of patients dying of a variety of diseases into the vaginas or uteruses of rabbits with a brush or syringe shortly after delivery. Seven of the nine experiments resulted in the animal's death, and induced pathological changes that at autopsy were indistinguishable from those found in women dying of childbed fever. One healthy animal was sacrificed, and no gross pathological changes were seen at autopsy.

Semmelweis's purpose in conducting the Lautner experiments is clear from the following passage in his *Aetiology*:

> 'I repeat my claim that in respect to discovering the cause of the illness of patients, it is extremely valuable to show experimentally that injecting decaying matter into the vagina produces pyemia…' (SC, 198).

That this was Semmelweis's *sole* purpose in conducting the Lautner experiments is evident from the following response to Carl Braun:

> 'If Carl Braun admits that the autopsy establishes pyemia in the rabbit, then he has admitted all that we wish to show by these experiments, i.e. that childbed fever is the same disease which occurs in general wherever a decomposed matter is introduced into the circulation.' (SM, 741-742).

The only *valid* technical criticism of the Lautner experiments was that mothers were examined during labor, and, therefore, the causative agent introduced into their lower genital tracts *before* the placenta was delivered and any injuries during delivery could have been sustained—i.e. before sites of ingress into the blood stream were opened up—whereas in rabbits cadaveric particles were introduced *after* delivery. Semmelweis conceded the point, and in his response reaffirmed that all he intended to show with the Lautner experiments was that pyemia could be induced in rabbits and nothing more:

> 'If we have wholly neglected to introduce the deleterious matter before the cast [i.e. delivery] one cannot cover every aspect of the subject in nine experiments, and *the question has only to do with the fact whether injected deleterious matter brings on the same process in animals as is observed in human puerperae*, and there is certainly more of an analogy between recently delivered rabbits into which deleterious matter was introduced after a recent cast, and a parturient who is infected in the lying-in hospital, than between the same parturient and an anatomist, wounded during an autopsy…' (SM, 611)

And it was not disputed that the same pathological changes *were* induced in seven of the nine Lautner experiments as found at autopsy in mothers dying of childbed fever, for Skoda told the Academy of Sciences on October 18, 1849:

> It is barely necessary to mention that the changes encountered in the corpses of the rabbits were the same as that resulting from puerperal fever, and, in general, from pyemia in human corpses. (vGy, 45, Appendix A, p. 172).

The following 4-steps of Semmelweis's reasoning is the most unequivocal explanation Semmelweis gave of why he conducted the Lautner experiments:

> 1. 'in the case of Kolletschka, lymphangitis, phlebitis, peritonitis, pleurisy, etc., were caused by the introduction of cadaveric material into the circulation, and since the anatomic findings in Kolletschka and in patients dead of puerperal fever are identical, then we assume for puerperal fever the same productive cause;'
>
> 2. 'the presence of this cause was not difficult to demonstrate on the hands of the examiners' [because of the odour it caused];
>
> 3. 'if now, as the result of appropriate measures, whose purpose was to destroy the material causing childbed fever, the mortality, which formerly varied between 237 to 518 deaths per year, is reduced to 45 deaths per year—[these were the figures Wieger published on April 20, 1849]—and under these circumstances it would never do to again examine patients with unclean hands, **in order to have proof that the mortality increased thereby;**' (boldface added)
>
> 4. 'but if the same thing takes place in the experiments on animals…it is thus proven that the decomposed matter, clinging to the hands…causes the frequent morbidity among the puerperae in the First Obstetric Clinic.' (SM, 609).

In other words, Semmelweis was saying that having proved that he could prevent the disease he now wanted to prove that he could cause it, i.e. bring it about, and because he could not ethically prove this in humans, he proved it in animals.

Why Semmelweis delayed publishing his results

The most puzzling aspect of Semmelweis's story is why he did not publish the results of his research for eleven years. The vast literature on Semmelweis has offered only speculations, not answers to the puzzle, attributing his failure to publish sooner to psychological factors[64] or supposed inability to write,[65] and has claimed that it contributed significantly to his doctrine being misunderstood and rejected.[66] Lesky herself offered only contradictory statements. In her monograph, she suggested, '[h]ere it becomes completely clear how disastrous Semmelweis's reluctance to publish was for …the dissemination of his doctrine,' [**M, 85**], but in her *magnum opus* the following year, she drew an entirely different conclusion:

> 'Thus, it may be said that hardly any [medical] discovery had ever received such quick publicity as that by Ignaz Semmelweis. It is only legend therefore if the delayed acceptance of Semmelweis's theory is constantly ascribed to the fact that Semmelweis himself tarried writing about it. In order to arrive at the true reason, it has to be borne in mind that Semmelweis discovery required a complete reversal in the approach to the entire theory of "fevers" which at the time formed the greater part of the contemporary nosology.' (Lesky, 187)

It is also only 'legend' that Semmelweis had difficulty with the written word or could not write in the manner of an educated man. Carter

---

[64] Loudon, p.100 (Semmelweis's supposed intolerance of criticism); Dunn (2005) (Semmelweis's supposed inferiority complex because 'of his Hungarian origin and provincial German accent', an unsupported speculation Dunn took from Nuland (2003), p. 173).

[65] Sinclair, p. 8 (speculating about Semmelweis's inability 'to write with facility in the style of an educated man', but admitting that this was 'based on by no means conclusive evidence); Nuland (2003), p 174, (asserting that Semmelweis 'felt unqualified to write'); Obenchain, p. 115 (asserting that Semmelweis had 'trouble with the written word').

[66] Loudon, p. 100.

noted in the preface to his translation of Semmelweis's *Aetiology* that "the original edition of *Aetiology* is much better written than most scholars seem to believe," (SC, p. ix), and Gillies concluded that Semmelweis "stated his views clearly, and often developed incisive arguments in their favour."[67] To this may added that Semmelweis often wrote with wit—'Naturally, one cannot have much positive understanding of that which does not exist,' (SC, 204); irony—'victims are depicted as dissipated and yet assumed to possess such tender modesty as never appears in the higher classes,' (SC 160); and sardonic humor, as in the following concerning Braun and Scanzoni's theories about the cause of childbed fever:

> 'And how competent Braun is to discuss the etiology of childbed fever is shown by the fact that he has puerperal fever begin without demonstrable changes and leave off without ascertainable causes, although 30 causes of childbed fever are known to him. Scanzoni at least lets the puepera die from puerperal fever only in part from unascertainable causes; for rest he has a more certain etiological factor for childbed fever in change.' (SM, 738)

But Semmelweis could also express himself with extraordinary lyricism, as in this comment on the discussions of childbed fever at the Paris Academy in 1858:

> but the dry straw, which therein was brought to light, we shall leave unthreshed since there is no grain to be beaten out of it; (SM, 704)

Or in this on the Prague maternity hospital:

> the sorrowful humanitarian can estimate what a horrible waste of human life took place also in the Prague lying-in hospital. (SM, 600).

And he could certainly write with sophistication, as in this reply to Braun:

> 'Braun has reproached me because I depend on the past, and draw therefrom very bold conclusions...Into what barbarity

---

[67] Gillies (2005), p. 169.

> would humanity sink, if the past were lost for the succeeding generations. Can a generation discovery navigation and build a great Eastern? How many generations have labored until one contrived the locomotive, which could climb the Semmering?...Braun may scarcely remember how much he looked about the past as he was compiling his textbook of Obstetrics. For of a surety I am convinced that, if we strike out of this textbook everything which has to do with the past, nothing but the cover will be left which has to do with the present.' (SM, 740)

Semmelweis said of himself that he was averse to controversy and had "an innate aversion to every form of writing," (SM, 352), and there is no reason to doubt that what he said was true, but it still does not explain why he did not publish his results in a medical journal *sooner*: after all, Semmelweis *did* publish his results and was, once he put pen to paper, quite a prolific writer.[68] Moreover, we do not have conscious insight into the reasons for our own actions, and the accounts we give of them are often post hoc rationalizations.[69]

The first obvious reason that Semmelweis did not rush to publish his results at the end of 1847 was that there was a recrudescence of the

---

[68] Kadar (2020). (In addition to writing letters to the heads of maternity clinics around Europe after he first obtained the results of the chlorine hand-disinfection experiment,(SM, 565), Semmelweis wrote letters to the Academie des Science in Paris (Wieger, p. 398), to Wieger and Stolz in Strasbourg, (SM, 451), Levy in Coppenhagen, (SM, 584), and Everken in Paderborn, (SM, 711) concerning his theory, as well as two letters in English, one to the London Medical Times and Gazette, (Murphy (1946), p. 667. Semmelweis also published a case report in 1857, (vGy, 541-543), the year the Hungarian medical journal, *Orvosi Hetilap* (Medical Weekly), resumed publishing in June 1857 (S, 131)); the following year (1858) he published seven articles on childbed fever, (vGy, 61-83, Murphy (1946), pp. 663-664), and the next year wrote an article (published in 1860) explaining the difference between his doctrine and that of the English 'contagionists'. (vGy, 88-94). Finally, after he published his *Aetiology*, his controversial 'Open Letters' letters to critics of his doctrine, (vGy, 465-511), and a report on the discussion of the etiology and prophylaxis of childbed fever by the St. Petersburg Medical Society, (vGy, 512-537), never to write on the topic of childbed fever again, Semmelweis wrote five articles on gynecologic surgery during the period 1862-1865, the last one on ovariotomy remaining unpublished at the time of his death on August 13, 1865. (vGy, 543-597).

[69] Timothy D. Wilson, Strangers to Ourselves, Chapter 5, Knowing Why, Harvard University Press (2002), pp. 93-115.

disease after chlorine hand-disinfection was implemented. Although Semmelweis quickly deduced the reasons for the increase in MMR, there is clear evidence that he realized that he needed more follow up to convince others, and could not rush to publish his results in December, 1847, when Hebra publicized the discovery in an Editorial in the Journal of the Society of Physicians. (SM, 561-562).

Given how tenaciously he insinuated himself into Semmelweis's research, Skoda was likely the one pressing for the announcement, (vGy, 40, Appendix A, p167—'Sometime after Dr. Semmelweis had applied the chlorinewash with apparent favorable results, Professor Rokitansky, myself, and other physicians in the hospital reported his idea'), and since the Editorial contained statements that Semmelweis would surely have corrected—e.g. that putrid substances had injurious consequences even on *unwounded* skin—Gortvay and Zoltán concluded that Semmelweis did not see the Editorial before it was published, and may not even have known that it was going to be published. (G-Z, 59) Moreover, Hebra did not report the actual results of the chlorine hand-disinfection experiment: he published only two unrepresentative averages showing that chlorine hand-disinfection had reduced the MMR on the first maternity clinic from 18% to 2.75%. (SM, 561-562) Hebra also took the unusual step of asking 'directors of obstetrical institutions' to report 'confirming or disconfirming results to the editors of this journal' (Ibid., and not Semmelweis, it should be noted), and which may reflect that Semmelweis's supporters realized that the evidence was not yet sufficiently persuasive.

That Semmelweis and the young doctors visiting him at the time perceived the need for further follow up is evident from the letter that Routh wrote to Semmelweis after Routh left Vienna at the end of December, 1847 (vGy, 33):

> 'Do you think that the cases which occurred after my departure also support your opinions? Is childbed fever less common than before? If this dangerous disease occurs less frequently in the obstetrical wards than formerly, then this most significant success is established.' (SM, 566-567)

That Semmelweis also perceived the need for further follow up is evident from the following reply to Scanzoni, who claimed that he had tried chlorine hand-disinfection in Prague, but it was ineffective:

> 'About the middle of May we introduced the chlorine washings, and thereupon the mortality decreased to 6 deaths in June, to three in July, to five in August, but in September rose again to 12, in October to 11, in November to 11, and in December to eight. *From this increased mortality in spite of the chlorine washings* we did not draw the conclusion that they were futile, but the increased mortality raised in us the suspicion that, perhaps in spite of the chlorine washings, decomposed matter was being introduced into the patients, and an investigation made for this reason showed that some of the students were slighting the chlorine washings. We found that after the examination of a parturient suffering from a cancer of the uterus we did not wash our hands in chlorine of lime, just as we did not isolate the woman with the carious knee...; for these reasons we did not abandon the chlorine washings, but on the contrary, we practiced them even more assiduously, with the happy result that during seven months of 1848 we lost less than one of 100 puerperae...' (SM, 602, italcs added).

But, as already noted, there was another reason Semmelweis did not publish his results as soon as he had sufficient follow up: his conclusion that the results of the hand-disinfection experiment proved his theory of causation was rejected by Klein and others at the AKH, and he wanted to meet this objection before publishing his result. Although Semmelweis felt the Lautner experiments had countered this objection, Skoda, unfortunately, believed otherwise, and told the Academy of Sciences that the Lautner experiments had not resolved the doubts about Semmelweis's theory, and that 'further and more varied' animal experiments were required to resolve them. Semmelweis conducted these experiments with Brücke in the spring and summer of 1850, but they yielded ambiguous results, and Brücke concluded that only further clinical observations could resolve the doubts about Semmelweis's theory, which Semmelweis was not a position to make in Vienna as his request for an extension of his assistantship had been denied. That is the most likely reason Semmelweis did not publish his results before he left Vienna and returned to Pest in October, 1850.[70] Moreover, after he returned to Pest Semmelweis was still not in a position to acquire the further clinical observations that Brücke had said was needed to remove any remaining doubts about Semmelweis's theory for another six years.

Semmelweis took an unpaid position as Director of the Obstetric Division of St. Rókus Hospital on May 20, 1851, but the hospital did not have enough deliveries for him to acquire sufficient clinical data for a number of years as it admitted obstetrical patients only during the months of August and September, when the university was on vacation. During the rest of the year, the obstetrical beds were filled with surgical patients. But as soon as Semmelweis did have sufficient evidence to report—which was within a year of him being appointed Professor at the University of Pest— he allowed his assistant to report the results of chlorine hand-disinfection at the university hospital only the report was greeted with a derisory editorial comment, as previously described:

> 'We thought this theory of chlorine disinfection had died out long ago: the experience and statistical evidence of most of the lying-in institutions protest against the opinions expressed in this article: it would be well that our readers should not allow themselves to be misled by this theory at the present time.' (S,127)

Never the less, Semmelweis acquired important evidence that corroborated his theory at St. Rókus Hospital. Indeed, at the very first medical meeting Semmelweis attended in Pest his theory was challenged with the fact that St. Rókus Hospital was plagued with epidemics of childbed fever and yet no medical students were taught at that hospital, nor were autopsies performed routinely there—the chief of surgery performed only forensic autopsies and only sporadically. (SM, 413) Semmelweis visited the hospital the next day and immediately understood the reason for the epidemics: the cause was the same as the cause of the 'row infections' on the first maternity division in Vienna after the admission of the mother with carcinoma of the uterus.

---

[70] Kadar (2020).

The chief of surgery was in charge of obstetrics at Rókus Hospital, and he made ward rounds on women in labour after he had made ward rounds on his surgical patients, most of whom had wound infections and purulent discharges, and contaminated the surgeon's hands with decaying matter. (SC, 106-107). Over the first five years as Chief of Obstetrics at the hospital, Semmelweis reduced the annual MMR from childbed fever at the hospital to 0.85% by chlorine hand-disinfection, (SC, 108), thus refuting the first challenge to his theory, and confirming the non-cadaverous source of the causative agent.

The university hospital in Pest was also plagued by 'epidemics' of childbed fever. After assuming his post as Professor of Obstetrics at the University, and implementing chlorine hand-disinfection, Semmelweis had reduced the MMR from childbed fever to 0.39% by the end of his first year, as previously noted, but after a while there was a recrudescence of the disease. This time Semmelweis was able to track down the cause from the fact that none of the babies of the mothers who had suddenly contracted childbed fever had died after birth. Semmelweis inferred from this that the mothers must have contracted the infection after delivery otherwise their babies would also have been infected, and traced the cause of the infection to poorly washed bed linen. (SM, 428) This was further confirmation of the correctness of his theory of the cause and pathogenesis of childbed fever.

Since Fleischer's report received such a hostile reception in Vienna, it was understandable that Semmelweis would be reluctant to try to publish any further data in a Viennese medical journal, but there were no Hungarian medical journals being published when Semmelweis returned to Pest. Semmelweis had returned to a defeated country under martial law,[71] run by German-speaking officials, including the Austrian gendarmerie, who had replaced the local police and sent spies to all scientific meetings to ferret out political conspiracies, and required the minutes of every meeting to be submitted to the authorities. The Hungarian

[71] Taylor, p. 85. (Hungary's War of Independence ended on August 13, 1849, when Hungary surrendered to the joint forces of Russia and Austria at Világos; less than two months later, on the order of the Tsar, thirteen Hungarian generals and the former Prime Minister, Batthyányi were executed on October 6, 1849.)

Academy of Sciences had suspended its meetings, the only Hungarian medical journal had ceased publication, and the only medical publication in Hungary was the officially censored Minutes of the Pest Medical Society. (S, 118-119) Only when Martial law was lifted in 1854, and amnesty declared in 1856, was there a revival of intellectual life in Pest. (S, 130-131) The leader of the revival, Janos Balassa, Professor of Surgery at the University, started a weekly medical journal called the *Medical Weekly* (*Orvosi Hetilap*) edited by Lajos Markusovszky, Semmelweis' close friend from their student days in Vienna, which began publishing in June, 1857, and Semmelweis submitted a case report that same year. (vGy, 541-543) Starting in January, 1858, Semmelweis delivered four lectures on his doctrine to the Medical Society of Pest-Buda that were published in the *Medical Weekly*. (vGy, 61-83) Semmelweis started writing his *Aetiology* the following year, completed it in August 1860, and it was published two months later (although for unknown reasons the year of publication on the title page is 1861). The German medical historian Georg Stickler ranked Semmelweis's book "with the classics of medical literature, in line with Robert Koch's *Investigations on the Aetiology of Wound-Infection* and Pasteur's *Chicken Cholera.*" (G-Z, 154).

Summary

The documents Lesky discovered and published in her monograph chronicle the depth of support Semmelweis enjoyed from progressive members of the Vienna Medical School, but they also revealed that despite his conservatism and doubts about Semmelweis's theory, Klein took Semmelweis theory seriously, and permitted him to implement what must have been a fairly disruptive new undertaking—chlorine hand-disinfection by attendants before entering the labor ward. Moreover, Klein allowed Semmelweis to continue with the hand-disinfection despite the resurgence of childbed fever after the summer of 1847, and to make it even more intrusive by requiring attendants to disinfect their hands before examining any patient on the labor ward, and not only before entering the labor ward.

Klein continued to harbor reservations about Semmelweis's theory even after the evidence of the effectiveness of the chlorine hand-disinfection had become very persuasive towards the end of 1848. These reservations—that just because the MMR from childbed fever fell after chlorine hand-disinfection was implemented, it did not necessary mean that the hand-disinfection had caused the MMR to fall, especially not as the incidence of childbed fever was known to fluctuate widely—were shared by others both inside and outside Vienna and the AKH. Nevertheless, Klein was amendable to extending Semmelweis's assistantship so that he might continue his research, and gave Semmelweis a good reference on November 19, 1848, less than three weeks after fresh riots in Vienna were suppressed by Field Marshall Windish-Grätz after laying siege to Vienna and five days of bloody fighting that began on October 26, 1848. This seems remarkable given that Klein was said not to like foreigners, Semmelweis was Hungarian, and the October riots were triggered by the Emperor's sending of troops to quell the Hungarian uprising. But everything changed after Skoda injected himself into Semmelweis's research—never having previously shown any concern at the carnage childbed fever was causing on the first maternity clinic so far as is known.

Klein had no objection to the appointment of a commission or to an investigation into the cause of the fall in MMR from childbed fever on his department after chlorine hand-disinfection was implemented. Klein objected to Skoda's proposal only after he was excluded from the commission selected to conduct the investigation, and changed his mind about extending Semmelweis's assistantship because with Skoda's motion the research was threatening to create what amounts to a hostile work environment. But this was far from the end of the matter, or the end of Skoda's involvement in Semmelweis's research.

Other documents indicate that starting three days after his assistantship ended Semmelweis conducted experiments in nine domestic rabbits over a five-month period with Launter, and successfully induced pathological changes in seven of the nine animals indistinguishable from those found in mothers dying of childbed fever. Semmelweis conducted these experiments for the express purpose of demonstrating that what he postulated was the cause of childbed fever could induce pathological changes characteristic of childbed fever in animals. However, two months after the last experiment ended, Skoda delivered a lecture before the

Imperial Academy of Sciences in which he gave an inaccurate account of how Semmelweis was led to his discovery—inaccurate as judged by Semmelweis's own account, that is—and stated that the animal experiments Semmelweis had conducted with Lautner had failed to resolve the doubts about Semmelweis's theory they were intended to resolve. He also asked the Academy to award Semmelweis a grant to conduct further and more varied animal experiments, only this time to conduct them with Brücke, a member of the Academy, to ensure that they were conducted properly. Semmelweis conducted these additional experiments with Brücke in the spring and summer of 1850, but they yielded only ambiguous results, which led Brücke, the leading physiologist of his day, to conclude that only further clinical observations, not animal experiments, could resolve any remaining doubts about Semmelweis's theory of the cause of childbed fever.

All the while, Semmelweis successfully applied for his 'habilitation,' but his application for a docentur, with permission to teach on cadavers as well as manikins, was denied. He reapplied for a docentur on May 9, 1850, and agreed provisionally to limit his request to teaching on manikins until the 'cadaver question' was decided in the reasonable hope that the question would be resolved in his favor given that Rokitansky was by then Dean of the Medical School, and Rokitansky supported the use of cadavers for teaching by private docents. However, Rokitanky was unsuccessful in getting the regulations changed, and Semmelweis was granted a docentur that limited him to using only leather manikins for teaching. Semmelweis, therefore, left Vienna and returned to Pest in October, 1850, because the docentur would not have allowed him to issue certificates of satisfactory attendance and completion to student who took his course.

The same information, except that contained in Schwartz's letter to Michaelis, was available to Lesky, but she constructed a very different narrative of what happened to Semmelweis in Vienna from that same information. Her narrative portrayed Skoda, 'the main campaigner,' and other progressive members of the Vienna Medical School as waging a relentless battle against a conservative, authoritarian bureaucracy on behalf of Semmelweis and his discovery in which only Semmelweis did not pull his weight by failing to write up his research, and by abruptly leaving Vienna in October, 1850. Her narrative rejected Semmelweis's own account of his discovery *tout court*, and accepted instead Skoda's account of the discovery based on Podach's historically unsupportable speculation that Semmelweis's account was likely an after-the-fact reconstruction.

Lesky viewed Skoda's motion to the medical College of Professors that turned Klein against Semmelweis and cost Semmelweis his job, as the first offensive in this unrelenting battle fought on behalf of Semmelweis's discovery. She declared Skoda's lecture to the Academy of Sciences, in which Skoda told the Academy that doubts still remained about Semmelweis's theory—because the animal experiments Semmelweis had conducted with Lautner had failed to resolve those doubts—as the opening of a new offensive on behalf of Semmelweis after the first offensive failed, and disregarded what Brücke had told the Academy of Sciences about the additional animal experiments that Semmelweis conducted with Brücke at Skoda behest to resolve these remaining doubts. Lesky construed Semmelweis's lecture to the Society of Physicians as the first victory of the progressive wing of the Vienna Medical School against their and Semmelweis's enemies. She then declared the award of a docentur to Semmelweis that limited him to teaching on leather manikins as the first victory of the Vienna Medical School against the Ministry of Education, and Semmelweis's departure from Vienna shortly thereafter as 'incomprehensible,' notwithstanding that Rokitanky failed to get the regulations pertaining to the use cadavers for teaching by private docents changed. Lesky concluded her narrative by implying that but for the fact the Semmelweis had not published his research, his supporters would have succeeded in having Semmelweis appointed to succeed Klein as professor of the first maternity division of the AKH following Klein's death in 1856.

Discussion

What then should one make of Lesky's narrative in the light of this critique? Given how critical Lesky was of Schürer von Waldheim's disregard and uncritical use of historical material, the most striking aspect of Lesky's narrative is her own disregard and uncritical treatment of the historical material available to her. Documents and the information they contain do not come ready-made as evidence: they become 'evidence' only if they are used to infer answers to historical questions about the past, and only if the inferential inquiry is conducted in a certain way. As Oakeshott put it:

> 'A historically understood past is the conclusion of a critical enquiry **of a certain sort**, inferred from circumstantial evidence, a past that is composed of passages of related events...but to be a passage of historical past, the relationship must be **of a certain kind**, namely, between antecedent and subsequent events in terms of which we come to understand what in fact they are historically.
>
> This does not mean that every event is related in this way to every other event, but only that no historical event is without a significant relationship with some other historical event. However, mere antecedence is not in itself a significant relationship. Therefore, an historical enquiry must distinguish between antecedent events, and detect which are significantly related to the subsequent, and thereby transform the subsequent into some kind of a consequent.'[72]

In other words, to understand the past *historically* is to understand the contingent relationship between events, but this can only be understood if a certain kind of inquiry is conducted, and this is precisely the kind of inquiry that Lesky did not conduct.

For example, Lesky disregarded the animal experiments that Semmelweis conducted with Lautner and Brücke. She ignored Skoda's conclusions about the Lautner experiments; she ignored Brücke's conclusions about the fresh set of experiments Semmelweis conducted with Brücke at Skoda's behest; and, therefore, Lesky was oblivious to how Semmelweis might have construed the fact that two such academically respected and prominent individuals believed that Semmelweis had not resolved the doubts about his theory with his animal experiments. But the most significant event Lesky elided as far as Semmelweis's discovery, and

[72] Oakeshott (1999/1983), pp. 36, 76-78 (boldface added).

the role that Kolletschka's death played in the discovery were concerned, was Semmelweis's extensive autopsy experience that spanned more than two years by the time of Kolletschka died on March 13, 1847. Lesky readily acknowledged Semmelweis's pathological experience with respect to gynecological diagnoses and his failure to publish on his work in that field, but not his autopsy experience with respect to childbed fever as that enabled her to credit Podach's historically unsupportable speculations about Semmelweis's account of the role that Kolletschka's death played in his discovery.

And even when Lesky did connect events, she declined to interpret subsequent events as consequences of contingently-related antecedent events if the connection did not fit her narrative. So, for example, she viewed Skoda's motion to the College of Professors as inextricably linked to Semmelweis's request for a two-year extension of his assistantship, and, therefore, absolved Skoda of any responsibility for the consequences that his motion had on Semmelweis's career in Vienna. This link was entirely notional, and supported only by the convoluted and conclusory argument that (1) the medical faculty had a moral obligation to expand medical knowledge; (2) this moral obligation compelled the medical faculty to conduct the kind of investigation into Semmelweis's discovery Skoda was proposing; and (3) the proposal was bound to embroil Semmelweis's application for an extension in a power struggle between the medical faculty and the Ministry of Education over who was authorized to make decisions on educational matters. And the link did not explain why the obligation to expand medical knowledge required a commission to do precisely what Semmelweis had wanted to do, and requested an extension of his assistantship to enable him to do it: continue his research so as to resolve any remaining doubts about his theory.

Still, it has been claimed that

> 'Historical interpretations differ even when the experts agree on the facts [and the] only safe generalization about history is still that it is being, and always will be rewritten, not only because new facts come to light, but because every age, and every historian, looks upon the past from a different perspective.'[73]

[73] Meyerhoff, p. 21.

So the question boils down to whether the narratives in Lesky's monograph and the critique of it are simply two very different but equally valid accounts of the same events separated by more than half a century, 'like two views of the same landscape seen from two different points,'[74] or whether it can be said that one is in some sense more veridical than the other? These questions go to the heart of what has concerned and continues to concern philosophers about what they see as the relativity of history and the impossibility of objective historical knowledge:

> 'no historian can describe the past as it actually was…every historian's work—that is, his selection of facts, his emphasis, his omissions, his organization, his method of presentation—bears a relation to his own personality and the age and circumstances in which he lives.'[75]

The difficulty stems from the fact that we cannot know and understand the past in the same way as we know and understand the natural world.[76] Therefore, we cannot explain historical events in the same way as we explain natural event, 'by subsuming what is to be explained under a general law.'[77] We can acquire knowledge of the 'laws of nature' by inductive inferences from observations. We can construct models to account for natural phenomena, and test our models by reproducing events under controlled conditions, i.e. experimentation, or by showing that future happenstance occurrences agree with what our models would have predicted. But we cannot obtain knowledge of the past or explain past events in the same way because the past is not an ontologically real past. What 'actually happened in the past cannot be found, nor dug up, nor retrieved, nor collected but only inferred.'[78] We cannot recreate the past as it was or verify our constructions of the past either by experimentation or by showing that similar events occurred under like conditions at other times and places, for the laws of nature that allow us to link similar occurrences have no parallel in history. 'Every judgment that we

---

[74] Popper, p. 302.
[75] Meyerhoff, p. 139..
[76] Berlin, pp. 19-20.
[77] Dray, p. 1.
[78] Oakeshott (1999), p. 36.

formulate, whether in historical thought or ordinary life, involves general ideas and propositions without which there can be no thought or language,'[79] but there are no 'laws of history.'

The evidence used to answer questions about the past is also always incomplete, and there are always gaps in our knowledge. These gaps in the historical evidence are filled in by interpolations that are both constructive and imaginative, and not by deductive or inductive inferences. But this does not necessarily make an account of the past relative or subjective or speculative. For example, Semmelweis's application for an extension of his assistantship, has not survived; what has survived is a document indicating that he made the application on December 1, 1848, and a letter by Klein to the Ministry of Education explaining why Klein had denied Semmelweis's application to which Klein attached a supplement stating that on November 19, 1848 he had given Semmelweis a very favorable reference. From this evidence, Lesky concluded that the purpose of the favorable reference Klein gave Semmelweis on November 19, 1848 must have been to support the application for an extension of his assistantship that Semmelweis made on December 1, 1848, which in turn must have meant that Klein was amenable to extending Semmelweis's assistantship before Skoda made his proposal to the medical College of Professors on January 16, 1849. The logic of this filling in of gaps in the historical evidence is different from the logic of inductive or deductive inference: Collingwood called it historical imagination. 'What is imagined is neither real nor unreal,' and, therefore, we obviously cannot 'prove' that Semmelweis used the reference to support his application, or that Klein was amenable to extending his assistantship, but we can show that the evidence constrains us to believe Lesky's conclusions, and that her conclusions are not illusory but something we are forced by the evidence to accept.

The core concept of what a *historical* construction of the past requires is expressed in Collingwood's theory of 're-enactment.' The subject matter of history is different from the subject matter of natural science in that it largely involves the actions of human beings. Therefore, the historian is concerned with discovering not merely events but the

---

[79] Berlin, p. 47.

thoughts expressed in those events, and to do this historians have to put themselves in the position of the historical actor, and rethink for themselves what the actor thought about the situation, and the possible ways of dealing with it:

> 'This re-enactment is only accomplished...so far as the historian brings to bear on the problem all the powers of his own mind and all his knowledge...It is not a passive surrender to the spell of another's mind; it is a labor of active and therefore critical thinking. The historian not only re-enacts past thought, he re-enacts it in the context of his own knowledge and therefore in re-enacting it criticizes it, forms his own value, corrects whatever error he can discern.'[80]

This is not a methodological prescription; it is a statement of what is required to understand not only the 'what' and 'when' and 'how' but also the 'why' of past events, and the essence of that requirement is empathy with the historical actor.

> 'To understand a human action...it is necessary for the inquirer somehow to discover its 'thought-side;' it is not sufficient merely to know the pattern of overt behavior. The historian must *penetrate* behind appearances, achieve *insight* into the situation, *identify* himself sympathetically with the protagonist, *project* himself imaginatively into the situation. He must *revive, re-enact, rethink, re-experience* the hopes, fears, plans, desires, views, intentions, etc., of those he seeks to understand.'[81] (italics in original)

Herbert Butterfield construed the historian's task in exactly the same way:

> 'The story cannot be told correctly unless we see the personalities from the inside, feeling with them as an actor might feel the part he is playing—thinking their thoughts all over again and sitting in the position not of the observer but of the doer of action. If it is argued that this is impossible—and indeed it is—not merely does it still remain the thing to aspire

---

[80] Collingwood (1993), p. 215

[81] Dray, p. 119.

> to, but in any case the historian must put himself in the place of the historical personage, must feel his predicament, must think as though he were that man. Without this art not only is it impossible to tell the story correctly but it is impossible to interpret the very documents on which the reconstruction depends.'[82]

These accounts fairly describe the mental process by which Lesky must have interpreted Skoda's actions to conclude that

> 'Skoda, with the inner evidence of spiritual co-authorship, immediately recognized in this new, genuine product of those methods of investigation and thought that Rokitansky and he had so distinctly imprinted on their school…[and] felt, to the highest degree, responsible to science and humanity, to ensure that this intellectual property of the Viennese school took its place in science and obstetrical practice.' **[M, 61]**

Lesky's empathized with Skoda—he was the hero of her story; but Lesky was never able to put herself in Semmelweis's shoes, and interpret Semmelweis's actions from Semmelweis's perspective. That is why she disregarded Semmelweis's animal experiments, and what Skoda and Brücke told the Academy of Sciences about those experiments; and that is why she found it incomprehensible that, for example, Semmelweis did not use his theory of childbed fever as the primary support for his habilitation. But this becomes readily understandable if one puts oneself in Semmelweis's position, and rethinks the possible ways Semmelweis could have thought of dealing with the situation, as he could reasonably have concluded that to use his theory of childbed fever as the main support for his habilitation would only invite the same expressions of doubt about his theory that Skoda had raised before the Academy of Sciences. Whether this is actually why Semmelweis did not use his theory of childbed fever as his *habilitation* thesis cannot be known. We can, however, conclude that the antecedent facts that Lesky disregarded do provide a rational explanation for what was otherwise an incomprehensible action, and,

---

[82] Quoted by Dray, p. 119.

therefore, that Semmelweis's actions do have a rational explanation, even if Lesky chose not to search for one.

Admittedly, it could still be argued that to accept a rational explanation is not something rooted in evidence, but merely reflects a preference for rational over irrational behavior, and exemplifies the very subjectivity that has concerned philosophers about history. It is true that we impute rationality to human action where this can be identified because human beings are rational creatures, and we prefer rational explanations for actions to irrational actions as it allows us to understand them. But to conclude from this that historical constructions of the past are necessarily subjective because the accounts selected are always the ones historians prefer is to misconstrue the rationale of the previously described historical inquiry that relates past events to each other as antecedents and subsequent.

Antecedent and subsequent events are related to one another in an *historical account* of the past as parts related to the whole, which means that the parts must cohere, and the historian examines the whole to determine if it makes sense. There is, of course, no 'law of history' that mandates that historical constructions of the past be intelligible: intelligibility merely identifies the relationship between antecedent and subsequent events as contingent, and contingency is the *sine qua non* of historical understanding and explanation. Without contingent relationship between events we have, not history but chronicle. And that is what Lesky's monograph is: a chronicle of events. Lesky did not construct her narrative from responses to a series of questions and answers about the documents she discovered in the Austrian archives; she did not try to understand the events she chronicled by linking them to relevant antecedents events; and that is why she could not explain the events she described, and repeatedly called Semmelweis's actions "incomprehensible."

It is undeniable, to return to the original question, that newly discovered information will cause historical narratives to be emended. The very documents Lesky discovered prove this for we first realized that, for example, Klein was actually very amenable to extending Semmelweis's assistantship before Skoda made his motion to the medical College of

Professors from the information contained in the documents Lesky brought to light. 'The enlargement of historical knowledge comes about mainly through finding how to use as evidence…facts which historians have hitherto thought of no value to them,'[83] and, therefore, it is equally true that new insights will also cause historical narratives to be revised. This is how Carter 'enlarged' our knowledge of Semmelweis's thinking by noting that Semmelweis was the first to define a disease in terms of its necessary cause instead of signs and symptoms, and that Skoda never accepted Semmelweis's theory of the cause of childbed fever.[84] But this only means that our knowledge and understanding of history continually develops as new information is brought to light just as does our knowledge and understanding of any empirical science such as medicine; it does not in any way evidence the ineluctable relativity of history or that historical narratives are necessarily subjective.

The only relevant new evidence that has surfaced since Lesky wrote her monograph is Schwartz's letter to Michaelis, and the only significance of that letter is that it establishes that Semmelweis and the young doctors around him were aware of the objections that were or could be raised against their interpretation of the results of the chlorine hand-disinfection experiment. But this could reasonably have been inferred without that letter from the documents Lesky herself discovered for it is difficult, indeed impossible to believe that Klein would not have communicated his view of why the MMR from childbed fever had fallen after chlorine hand-disinfection was implemented on one of his daily ward rounds with Semmelweis and the medical students. Therefore, newly discovered evidence cannot explain the different accounts in Lesky's monograph and the present critique of it.

The information contained in the Lesky documents and Schwartz's letter make it possible to understand Semmelweis's motivation for conducting animal experiments with Lautner; the opinions expressed in the text of Skoda's lecture and Brücke's memorandum to the Academy of the animal experiments Semmelweis had conducted, make it possible to understand Semmelweis's motivation for leaving Vienna and for

---

[83] Collingwood (1993), p. 247.

[84] Carter (1984).

delaying the publication of his results, but only if the right questions are asked about these documents, which, however, Lesky never asked.

But why did Lesky not inquire into the opinions that Skoda and Brücke had expressed about the animal experiments that Semmelweis had conducted? After all, she knew that both sets of experiments had been conducted; she knew why Klein did not accept Semmelweis's contention that the chlorine hand-disinfection experiment proved his theory; and she must have known what Skoda and Brücke had said about the experiments for to entertain that she did not would be inconsistent with the meticulousness that Lesky's historical scholarship was famous for. Her failure to ask these salient questions are likely explained by the first of the four factors that Walsh suggested 'actually make for disagreement among historians:' that is,

> 'the personal likes and dislikes [of the historian], whether for individuals or classes of persons. Historian A (Carlyle would be an example) admires great men; historian B (e.g. Wells) has a strong antipathy to them. Historian A, in consequence, makes his whole narrative centre around the ideas and actions of his hero…'[85]

Lesky's life's work was the history of the Vienna Medical School; the founders of the New Medical School, Skoda and Rokitansky, were brilliant men who supported Semmelweis, and nominated him to succeed Klein on Klein's death in 1856, six years after Semmelweis had returned to Pest. That these men should have played no part in what Lesky acknowledged was 'one of the greatest discoveries in the history of medicine' was simply inconsistent with Lesky's beliefs about the Vienna Medical School and its founders. She could not bring herself to acknowledge that credit for the discovery belonged to Semmelweis alone, much less that Skoda's use of Semmelweis's discovery for his own political ends, no matter how well-intentioned or high-minded it might have been, ended up destroying Semmelweis's career prospects in Vienna.

That is not to say that Lesky was necessarily conscious of this, the tendentiousness of her polemic notwithstanding. Beliefs must cohere if

[85] Walsh, p. 216.

they are to make sense of the world,[86] and conflicts between beliefs and facts are more often resolved, outside of conscious awareness, by interpreting facts to be consistent with beliefs rather than the other way around.[87] Lesky's statements (1) about Semmelweis most wanting to be Skoda's assistant when in fact he most wanted to be Kolletschka's assistant; (2) about Semmelweis's account of his discovery, and the pivotal role that Kolletschka's autopsy findings played in that discovery, being an after-the-fact reconstruction; and (3) about Semmelweis's use Skoda's *per exclusionem* method to deduce the cause of childbed fever, are all classic examples of confirmation bias that everyone uses to varying degrees to resolve conflicts between facts and beliefs, and that operates largely outside of conscious awareness.

Lesky resolved the conflict between the historical evidence and her beliefs about the Vienna Medical School and its founders by creating a narrative that was not an historical construction of the past at all, but what Butterfield called 'Whig history:' that is, the writing of history in the service of a present-day cause.[88] Lesky was forthright about the cause that her monograph was written to advance: to establish what Semmelweis's discovery owed to the Vienna Medical School, that the discovery was the intellectual property of the Vienna Medical School, and that Skoda was effectively its spiritual co-author. In advancing that cause, Lesky, *pari passu*, exonerated the Vienna Medical School from any responsibility for Semmelweis's fate in Vienna, and placed the blame solely on Semmelweis, the 'incomprehensible waverer' who refused to publish his results, and who 'escaped' from Vienna after being granted a position as private docent.

Oakeshott called such constructions of past events a *'practical'* past, as they are attempts to understand past events in relation to ourselves and our own current activities. These are very different constructions from an *historical* past understood in terms of contingently related antecedent events, but they are in fact the commonest kind of constructions of the past:

---

[86] Blackburn, pp. 17-28.
[87] Nickerson.
[88] Butterfield, pp. 30-31.

> 'Usually, we interpret these past happenings in relation to ourselves and our current activities. We read the past backwards from the present…we call upon the past to speak to us in utterances related to the present: and what appears is a practical past.'[89]

Therefore, Lesky is far from alone in using Semmelweis's discovery to explicate some topic of contemporary concern; she has much company from philosophers of science who have used Semmelweis's discovery to illustrate principles of inference and epistemological models so frequently that Scholl concluded that it had 'become a paradigm case of scientific discovery and confirmation within the philosophy of science.'[90] Indeed, Scholl, himself a philosopher of science, claimed that Semmelweis conducted the Lautner experiments to prove that 'cadaveric particles' when introduced into the lower genital tract could be absorbed into the blood stream, to answer the 'mechanistic question' left unanswered by considering clinical data in isolation.[91] However, since no one doubted that this could happen, because the sites of absorption were well known—the placental bed and any injuries to the lower genital tract sustained during delivery of the baby—this could not have been Semmelweis's purpose in conducting the Lautner experiments. That no one did actually doubt that 'cadaveric particles' introduced into the vagina could get absorbed into the blood stream is evident from following statements by Scanzoni about the Lautner experiments:

> 'as far as the inquiry into the cause of the frequent morbidity among puerperae is concerned, it is of no value to know that the injection of deleterious matter into the vagina may cause pyemia[92]—*knowledge of which incidentally did not require the experiments Dr. Semmelweis,* so highly valued by Professor Skoda, *as proof.*' (SM, 612, italics added).

---

[89] Oakeshott (1962), p. 162.
[90] Scholl, p. 67.
[91] Scholl, p. 75.
[92] Scanzoni considered the experiments 'of no value' because he did not accept that childbed fever was a form of pyemia.

Scholl's use of the past in this way is ironic, for Scholl acknowledged that philosophical debate of Semmelweis's discovery 'had neglected, to its detriment, historical facts.'[93] Lesky's narrative illustrates that philosophers have not been alone in neglecting historical facts to the detriment of our understanding of what really happened to Semmelweis in Vienna, and Lesky was certainly not the only historian to use Semmelweis's discovery in this way.[94]

Conclusions

The documents Lesky discovered in the Austrian Archives and published in her monograph have contributed information indispensable to understanding what happened to Semmelweis in Vienna, what immediate opposition his theory and proof faced from his chief and others at the AKH, why Semmelweis conducted animal experiments, and why he did not publish his work before leaving Vienna. However, Lesky constructed a narrative based on those and other already available documents that is not an historical account of Semmelweis's discovery because her narrative ignored the empirical observations, presuppositions and inferences on which that discovery was based and for which reliable evidence has survived. Lesky also elided other significant events for which reliable evidence has survived, such as Semmelweis's animal experiments, and what Skoda and Brücke had said about those experiments. Lesky ignored all this evidence because it was not relevant to the Whig history of Semmelweis and the Vienna Medical School she wanted to construct.

Lesky accepted Podach's speculations about Semmelweis's own account of his theory being an after-the-fact reconstruction uncritically, and used it to support her contention that Semmelweis deduced his theory of the cause of childbed fever by applying Skoda's method of differential diagnosis, which made Skoda effectively 'the spiritual co-author' of Semmelweis's discovery. However, Lesky failed to support her contention with historical evidence other than that Semmelweis had attended Skoda's lectures and clinic, and had applied to be Skoda's assistant after his

---

93 Scholl, p. 74.

94 Nuland (1979); Loudon, pp. 96-99.

application for Kolletschka's assistantship was unsuccessful. Although no biographer or historian has subsequently accepted Podach's speculations about Semmelweis's account of his own discovery being an after-the-fact reconstruction, Lesky's contention that Semmelweis's discovery was based on Skoda's *per exclusionem* method has stuck, and it has done a great disservice to the history of Semmelweis's discovery by erecting a barrier to a proper understanding of the depth of Semmelweis's reasoning, understanding and insights. This is regrettable.

APPENDIX A:

[36] Translation of Skoda's Lecture to the Academy of Sciences[95]

Joseph Skoda:

Regarding Dr. Semmelweis's Discovery of the True Cause of the Unusually High Incidence of Sickness among the Patients of the Viennese Maternity Hospital and the Means of Reducing This Incidence to Normal Levels

Lecture: held at the meeting of the Imperial Academy of Sciences on 18 October 1849 by a member in good standing

In the following, I believe that one of the most important discoveries in the field of medicine is the knowledge that Dr. Semmelweis, former assistant at the local Obstetrical clinic, brought to a venerated class, namely, discovery of the cause of the frequent sickening of women in this maternity clinic, and the means of reducing these sickenings to their usual number.

For the moment I will discuss the facts and conclusions from whose combination the discovery has arisen, and then report on the measures, which seemed necessary to put the discovery beyond doubt.

A. The combination of facts and conclusions from which the discovery took place can be combined in the following points:

1. For many decades, women sickened and died more often in the local obstetrical clinic than women outside the clinic, even though the care

[95] Page numbers in parenthesis refer to von Györy's compilation.

was better in the obstetrical clinic than is possible with country folk, and less wealthy citizens. While one observed the severest ravages of puerperal fever in the local obstetrical clinic, neither in Vienna nor in the countryside did one observe more frequent illnesses in women in the puerperium. This fact had to remove every thought of an epidemic directly producing puerperal fever. The more frequent sickening in the local obstetrical clinic, could not be considered a puerperal epidemic, regardless of the stereotypical contrary assertion.

2. Since a teaching department for doctors and a teaching department for midwives has existed in the local obstetrical clinic, the number of death specifically on the doctor's division until June, 1847 was constantly—in the year 1846 four times—higher than on the division for midwives as the following table shows **[37]**:

Year	Doctor's Division			Midwives' Division		
	No. Births	No. Deaths	No. Deaths per 100 Births	No. Births	No. Deaths	No. Deaths per 100 Births
1839	2781	151	5.4	2010	91	4.5
1840	2889	267	9.5	2073	55	2.6
1841	3036	237	7.7	2442	86	3.5
1842	3287	518	15.8	2659	202	7.5
1843	3060	274	8.9	2739	164	5.9
1844	3157	260	8.2	2956	68	2.3
1845	3492	241	6.8	3241	66	2.03
1846	4010	459	11.4	3754	105	2.7

It is understandable that such an enormous difference in mortality on two divisions of the same institution attracted general attention, and one sought to determine the root cause. The non-medical public required no particular ingenuity to discern that the views put forward by the doctors in official hearings were mistaken. In general, the most common view was that the medical treatment was to blame for the many deaths. In the process, one overlooked the fact that the medical treatment on the two divisions were no different.

A second opinion was that through the presence of younger men at childbirth injured female shame caused the sickening in the childbed, an opinion only the completely inexperienced can have. A further speculation recognized the bad reputation of the institution as the cause of the sickening, to which pregnant women were most unwilling to go, and to stay in which they constantly feared becoming ill. It is hardly necessary to notice that the bad reputation of the institution was first conditioned on the high mortality, that, therefore, this view did not take into account the start of the high rate of sickening. Furthermore, the representatives of this view can quickly convince themselves, if they look at the experience, that the sickening of recently delivered women has no connection to their fearfulness or timidity.

In the committee negotiations, the laundry, the confined space, and the unfortunate situation of the institution were blamed, although in all these respects the two **[38]** departments were the same. Understandably, the corresponding measures always remained without result. Towards the end of 1846, during discussions of a committee the opinion gained the upper hand that the sickening of recently delivered women was limited to obstetrical injuries that occur during teaching and examinations. But because midwives carry out such examinations in the same way, it was not prudent, in order to understand the more frequent illnesses on the department of physicians, to accuse the students, and especially the foreigners, that they are doing more rough examinations than the midwives. On this assumption the number of pupils was reduced from 42 to 20, the foreigners were almost completely excluded, and the examinations themselves reduced to the minimum.

The morality decline conspicuously in the months of December, 1846, January, February, and March, 1847; in April alone, despite the aforementioned measures, 57 died, in May 36 recently delivered women.

From that, the groundlessness of the above accusations of anyone became clear.

3. The Viennese school of anatomic pathology had established the following on the subject of puerperal illness:

The first organic abnormality to appear if a puerperal woman sickens is either-and to be precise most commonly - exudation at the wound on the inner surface of the uterus at the placental insertion site; or – less commonly – a partial or total conversion of the contents of a single or all the veins of the uterus to pus with previous or subsequent exudation from the vein walls; or, finally, an exudation on the peritoneum.

The just mentioned organic changes are followed after some time – sometimes very quickly – by the deposition of pus, or of a fibrous material, which soon turns into pus or liquid matter in various parts of the body, and occasionally complete jaundiced coloring of one part of the skin, whereby it represents a disease state—pyemia—build up of pus in blood.

From these facts the conclusion was drawn that pyemia in the puerperium as a rule develops from endometritis and uterine phlebitis. Thus, first caused are endometritis and uterine phlebitis.

Due to the rupture of veins during delivery, exposure of a large area of the uterine cavity, strain and other birth injuries, can quite easily explain the development of endometritis and uterine phlebitis. However, such an explanation is inconsistent with the highly unequal number of sickenings on the two division of the hospital. In the case of non-operative deliveries, the outcome on both departments must be the same. Now most deliveries are without operative intervention, so a history of lower operative procedures could cause though a small, not the stated enormous difference in the number of illnesses.

4. It is not uncommon for puerperae to experience intense fever as the first morbid phenomenon, and after a while **[39]** the symptoms of endometritis, inflammation of the uterine veins, peritonitis, and so on, come to the fore. In such cases, the exudate is sometimes at first purulent or ichorous, the exuding tissue softens, so that the morbid process right from the beginning represents a pyemia.

One is used to regard peculiar secretions of the mother as the predisposing, and an ordinary injury, for example, a cold or emotion, as the exciting cause of such diseases. Once again, such an assumption is inconsistent with the unequal number of illnesses on the two divisions.

5. Pyemia without prior suppuration or analogous suppurative changes in the organs arises from the action of rotting animal substance on the blood.—whether it is produced by other causes is unknown. As a rule, the rotting substance acts on the blood only through the wounded skin. After delivery, the uterine cavity presents a large wound surface; there are cracks in the cervix, and abrasions in the vagina. Putrefaction in the secretions of the uterus must therefore rarely have the effect of decaying matter on the blood, and, therefore, result in pyaemia.

The sickening of mothers from the putrefaction that develops in uterine or vaginal secretions under ordinary influences or the peculiar nature of the fluids of recently delivered women, could not account for the often mentioned unequal number of sickenings in the two departments. Moreover, it turned out that the violent fever, and then the uterine phlebitis, endometritis, etc., sometimes came on without the lochia becoming foul-smelling.

The question had to be raised whether in any way rotting or decaying substances could come into contact with the mothers' womb. After Dr. Semmelweis, as first assistant on the division of the Obstetrical institution intended for physicians, considered all the circumstances for a few months, he realized that both he and the students frequently examined corpses, that the cadaverous odor on their hands disappears only after a long time, despite washing several times, and that he and the students often crossing directly from the examination of the cadaver to the examination of the woman giving birth, was the only possible way of transferring a putrid animal substance to the birth site of the mothers. This was at the same time only one among the possible causes of puerperal disease, which on the division for midwives was either not at all effective or extremely limited, so that, assuming this cause, the very unequal number of diseases in the two departments would be very understandable. Midwives do not engage in autopsies, and the assistants for the midwife divisions seldom, because they only had midwives to deal with, rarely, seldom undertake autopsies. Also the decrease in sickening in the months of December, 1846, January, February, and March, 1847, as well as **[40]** the high mortality that occurred in April and May, agrees with the assumption that pathogenic potency derives from the autopsy room. The assistant of the maternity clinic rarely visited the autopsy room during the months of December, 1846, January, February, and March, 1847, for reasons that are not relevant here, the local students, moreover, whose number was reduced from 42 to 20, followed the assistant. Foreigners were firmly excluded from the maternity clinic. At the end of March, 1847, Dr. Semmelweis was assistant, and, partly for self-instruction, but primarily for the purpose of instructing the students, examined and practiced on corpses with unusual zeal.

Even without such a coincidence of circumstances, which confirm the hypothesis, Dr. Semmelweis had to think of means to remove the possible cause of the sickening of mothers.

This was not hard to find. Since exercises and examinations on corpses in medicine were essential, they had to be continued by the assistant and the students, so it was essential to remove every cadaverous atom from the hands before every examination. For this purpose, Dr. Semmelweis towards the end of May 1847 instructed everyone to wash his hands with chlorinated water before any examination of a pregnant woman, woman in labor or in the puerperium. Following this arrangement, puerperae on the student division suddenly sickened less numerously, the same as on the midwives' division. The number puerperae dying from then on was 6 in June, 3 in July, 5 in August, 12 in September, 11 in October, 11 in November, 8 in December. The year 1848 provided an even more propitious ratio. Namely, out of 3780 deliveries only 45 died: a ratio of 1.19 out of 100 [actually 1.21%]; while on the midwives' division out of 3219 deliveries 43 died: a ratio of 1.33 out of 100.

In the year 1849, up to the beginning of September, 60 puerperae died on the students' division and 76 on the midwives' division. This shows that from June, 1847 to the present, so already for a period of more than two years, while chlorinewashing was in use there was almost no difference in mortality on the two divisions of the obstetric clinic, whereas earlier over a seven year period the mortality on the students' division was three times as high as on the midwives' division.

B. I find the measures that seemed necessary, and that still seem necessary to put Dr. Semmelweis's discovery beyond all doubt, to be the following:

Sometime after Dr. Semmelweis had applied the chlorinewash with apparent favorable results, Professor Rokitansky, myself, and other physicians in the hospital reported his idea. We did not doubt for a moment that his view would be proved correct, and I did not hesitate to draw the attention of the Director of Medical Studies to the discovery in the **[41]** expectation that a commission could not fail to handle such an important topic. My report seems merely to have been noted. A reasonable prospect to bring clarity to the matter soon lay in the fact that in the Prague obstetrical clinic there were very numerous sickenings from time to time and to all appearances had the same causes as in Vienna. So I called for the introduction of chlorwashing in the Prague obstetric clinic.

In the negotiations in the Prague educational institution maintained in response to this call, the view that puerperal diseases are caused by epidemic influences prevailed, and it seems that chlorine washing has either not been applied at all, or not seriously.

Dr. Semmelweis wrote to several Professors of obstetrics abroad asking them to test his view of the cause of puerperal fever. A definite answer came only from the small obstetric clinic in Kiel. Dr. Michaelis reported on March 18, 1848, that the Board closed that institution on July 1, 1847 because of the high number of illnesses, and it remained closed until November. The illnesses began anew when the institution reopened, and he was thinking of closing it again when on December 21, he received notification of Dr. Semmelweis's discovery. Chlorwashing was immediately introduced, and since then only one illness occurred, and Dr. Michaelis thought that this followed use of a not well-sanitized catheter. On the other hand, Prof. Kiwisch in Würzburg, maintained that he not infrequently examined pregnant and laboring women immediately after making necropsies without observing any detrimental consequences.

After the year 1848, the Chairman of Studies of the College of Professors was entrusted with, and held that it was the duty of the Viennese medical Professors of the College to subject to a critical examination a discovery in Vienna of such great scientific and practical importance, and if the same was proved, to announce and acknowledge it. I, therefore, proposed to the College of Professors that it appoint a Commission to solve the following problems:

a) There is a table that gives the number of births and deaths, from month to month, as far as the dates go, and a list of the assistants and students in sequence, who assisted and practiced in the birth institution. Since 1828, while Professor Rokitancy had officiated on the pathology-anatomy division, one could find out, partly from his memory, partly from his autopsy logs, as well as through the memories of other physicians, if the involvement of assistants and students in autopsies was connected with the number of diseased individuals in the birth institution.

[42] b) To dig out the so-called 'street births.' There are births in the street, and their further care in Obstetrical institutions are not investigated except in cases in which the afterbirth has to be removed, or to treat a pathological obstetrical condition. If Dr. Semmelweis's opinion is correct, street births should become ill less often.

c) One must provide the precise number of births and deaths in all Obstetrical institutions within the Austrian empire, and, as far as possible, also from foreign ones, in order to determine if the mortality is less at all institutions where an infection cannot be acquired through cadaveric poison.

d) Finally, animal experiments should be undertaken.

The proposal was accepted by a majority of the College of Professors, and a Commission was immediately named; only the Ministry ruled on an objection from the Professor of Obstetrics, that a commission hearing should not take place. As a result of this decision, I asked Dr. Semmelweis that he himself undertake experiments in animals. If these are attained the other tasks are of less importance.

For the time being, rabbits were used for the experiments for several reasons.

> *First Experiment:* On March 22, discolored exudate from endometritis was introduced into the vagina and uterine cavity of a female with a moistened brush ¼ hour after delivery. The

animal was apparently quite well after that until on 24 April it was found dead.

Autopsy: The folded mucous membrane of the uterine horns is covered with a fluid, dirty gray exudate; some fluid in the left thoracic cavity; the lower lobe of the lung is covered with a coagulated, membranous pale-yellow exudate; its parenchyma, as well as that of the posterior lower third of the upper lobe of the lung, liver-like gray; the remainder of this lung, as well as the right lung, is air-filled and vermilion like. The heart is wrapped in a delicate, pale-yellow, villous exudate, and bathed in a few drops of liquid exudate.

Second experiment: On the 12th April, 12 hours after delivering a litter of 5, a female was treated in the same way as the first animal. Because the animal in the first experiments appeared quite well, it was believed that in the second animal the brush should be introduced one day after another for several days. On the 14th of April, the animal expressed pain when the brush was introduced, the uterus contracted violently, and expressed yellowish, white thick exudate. On 17th April, the animal was significantly ill, on the 22nd had diarrhea, and on the 23rd April the animal was found to be dead. The brush was introduced daily until death.

Autopsy: In the abdominal cavity, a few intestinal coils were bound together by a membranous, coagulated exudate; on the vaginal and uterine mucus membrane and tissues a rigid, yellow exudate; the uterine horns were moderately distended, and filled with **[43]** dirty-grey rotting exudate; in the colon there were several groups of ulcerating follicles, the mucus membrane was partly ulcerated, partly infiltrated with a yellow exudate, and each part surrounded by injected vessels. The lungs bright vermillion; in the left upper lobe there was a bean-sized bloody infiltrate with pus in the middle.

Third Experiment: On 15th April, a brush was introduced into a female for the first time some 10 hours after delivering a litter of four, and daily thereafter until death, which occurred on 21st April. On the 17th, the animal expressed pain at the introduction of the brush, and squeezed purulent exudate out of the uterus.

Autopsy: In the abdominal cavity, massive amount of liquid, and coagulated membranous exudate bound individual loops of bowel. The mucous membrane of the vagina and uterus were covered and infiltrated with a yellow, densely adherent exudate, the uterine horns were greatly distended with dirty, reddish-grey exudate. Lentil-size purulent exudates infiltrated the liver in several places, on the mucous membrane of the colon, near the appendix [Processus vermiformis]—larger than lentil-size ulcerated areas were covered with pale-yellow exudate and surrounded by injected vessels.

Fourth experiment: On the 24th of May, a brush dipped in diluted blood from a man who had died of marasmus 36 hours previously, was introduced into a strong female about an hour after delivering a litter of 5. On the 25th, a brush moistened with pleuritic exudate was introduced; on the 26th, with peritoneal exudate from a person with tuberculosis, and again on the 27th. From then on, the brush was not introduced any more. The animal appeared completely health, and on 24th of June delivered for a second time.

Fifth experiment: On 2nd June, a brush moistened with peritoneal exudate used in experiment 4 was introduced into a female about 12 hours after delivery. The introduction was repeated on the 2rd, 4th, and 5th of June, and after that the animal was left untouched. It appeared to remain healthy, and delivered again on June 28. On 29th of June, a brush freshly moistened in pleuritic fluid was introduced, and again on the 30th. The animal remained healthy, and on was killed on the 17th of July. Autopsy showed no changes indicative of pyemia.

Sixth experiment: On 10th of June, a brush moistened with purulent, pleuritic exudate from a male cadaver was introduced into a female several hours after delivery. From 11th to 30th of June, the peritoneal exudate of a man who had died of typhus was used to moisten the brush. The animal remained health, and delivered for a second time on July 13th. On the same day, the brush was freshly introduced, and from then on daily until the 24th of July. The animal became emaciated, developed diarrhoea, and died on 30th of July.

Autopsy: In the pericardium, drops of cloudy serum. Dirty-white, uneven, bumpy, pea-sized vegetarians could be felt sitting on the free edge of the top of the tricuspid valve, pushed into the conus arteriosus, intimately connected to the papillary muscles of the endocardium; the inner surface of the right ventricle is occupied by single, yellowish-white, nodular coagulum. In the peritoneal cavity, membranous coagulum and fluid exudate. In the periphery of the liver, and near the lower surface, a pea-sized infiltrate of firm, yellowish exudate.

The uterus is as in No. 4 procedure, only the infiltration and necrosis is still more considerable. Several veins of considerable thickness between the body of the uterus and the right horn were stuffed with firm yellow exudate.

Seventh Experiment: On 16th June, a brush moistened with pus from an abscess between the ribs of a man dead of cholera was introduced one hour after delivery. The brushing was performed daily until 3rd of July. The animal remained healthy and delivered on 18th July for a second time.

The experiment was then modified, and to avoid mechanical injury, a brush was no longer used. Fluid is brought into the genitalia by means of a triple syringe with a 3 inch long tube. Just after the injection, the animal **[181]** expressed the fluid. The injections were done daily until the 24th of July. The animal became emaciated, and found to be dead on 29th July.

[44] *Autopsy:* In both chest cavities some thick, yellow exudate; in the peritoneal cavity, two ounces of partly membranous, coagulated exudate; the uterus normal, pale, without exudate on its mucous membrane.

Eighth Experiment: On the 24th of June, the same animal was used as in the 4th experiment. The brushings occurred daily from 24th of June to 8th of July. The animal became severely emaciated, developed diarrhea, and was found dead on the 25th of June.

Autopsy: In the peritoneal cavity some yellow exudate; on the back wall of the uterus a thin layer of dirty yellow, intimately adherent exudate; in the horns of the same, some fluid, dirty,

> grey-red exudate; the border between the vagina and the uterus, corresponding to the junction of the urethra, was infiltrated with a bean-sized, purulent exudate, superficially necrotic in places; the ulcer formed with jagged undermined margins, the base covered with a layer of exudate, infiltrated an inch of the substance of the vagina with exudate.
>
> *Ninth Experiment:* On the 8th of August, peritoneal exudate from a man was injected a day after delivery. The animal immediately expelled the injected material. Injections were made daily for 15 days. The animal looked ill on the 13th, emaciated. On the 20th it was found dead.
>
> *Autopsy:* Some fluid exudate in the abdominal cavity; in the periphery of the liver, numerous, mostly hempseed-sized, yellow spots of inflammation. The mucous membrane on the back wall of the uterus was excoriated over the circumference of a lentil [*einer Linse excoriirt*]; the body was infiltrated with yellow exudate **[45]**on the peritoneum. The excoriation lay an inch higher as in [experiments] N. 6 and 8. The right uterine horn was infiltrated with such a great amount of exudate that it reached twice the volume of the free fluid on its mucous membrane, the veins in the broad ligament was filled with exudate.

It is barely necessary to mention that the changes encountered in the corpses of the rabbits were the same as that resulting from puerperal fever, and, in general, from pyemia in human corpses. One could object to the experiments just cited that in the process a greater quantity of putrefying matter was involved, and that the putrid substance in eight cases was brought into contact with the birth-parts of the animals for many days after each other, and once in only one case, whereas the quantity clinging to the hands—whatever it may be—must be considered very small, as the hands are always washed with water after examination of cadavers.

This objection seems to me to have no special weight, as, based on experience, the effect of the putrefying matter is on the blood, which is a consequence. The cause of wounding cannot depend on the quantity of putrid matter, which because of its smallness is hardly visible, as infection is not uncommonly caused by wounding. By the way, to remove any doubt, it seems expedient to conduct further and variously modified experiments in animals. Therefore, I ask that you be willing to support Dr. Semmelweis in further experiments with a grant of money, and in view of this, in order to dispel any doubts as to the correctness of the experiments, that these attempts are also made by a member of the Academy, I ask Professor Bruce to undertake this task.

The Section provisionally decided to allocate 100 guilders to Semmelweis, and at the same time expressed their inclination to approve larger sums if necessary. Professor Brücke was asked, simultaneously, to carry out the tests, which he has already agreed to do.

APPENDIX B:

Translation of Brücke's memorandum

Proceedings of the Imperial Academy of Sciences

Mathematics-Natural Science Section

Professor Brücke made the following notification:

Last autumn, at the request of Professor Skoda, this esteemed Section (*Classe*) asked me to conduct experiments in animals with Dr. Ignaz Semmelweis, in view of his statements about how puerperal fever came into being, and to that end gave us 100 florints. Dr. Semmelweis had already in the spring and summer made these attempts with great zeal and conscientiousness, and carried out the post-mortems on the animals with me. These have, however, until now delivered only ambiguous results, and have convinced me that experiments on animals are not the suitable means to lift the doubts about this important, and for everyone in whose eyes human life still has some value such an interesting topic, rather, that this can only happen through the collection of experiences similar to those Dr. Semmelweis made in the local obstetrical institution in a manner so pleasing to every humanitarian. In view of this, in agreement with Dr. Semmelweis, who had left Vienna during these days to pick up his residency in Pest, I herewith returned to the Imperial Academy of Sciences the instructions for 100 florins delivered to me on 31 October 1849.

APPENDIX C:

Translation of Minutes of Semmelweis's Lecture

Society of Physicians, May 15, 1850

Dr. Semmelweis, emeritus assistant on the first obstetrical clinic, developed his views on the genesis of puerperal fever; he shows numerically from the records that since 1839, since a special clinic for teaching obstetricians, and another for midwives, was set up, more than four times more women have died from puerperal fever on the first clinic than on the second, notwithstanding that admission of pregnant women between the two changed every 24 hours, from which he draws the simple conclusion that the increased incidence of puerperal fever on the first obstetric clinic could not be produced by general epidemic influences, but only locally, by endemic conditions.

Dr. Semmelweis then turned to endemic causes, as have been approached by others, such as the overcrowding of hospital rooms, the long-standing impregnation of the localities with puerperal miasma, the more frequent and supposedly rougher examinations of budding obstetricians, the pre-existing anxiety of pregnant women, and so on, in turn, and proved that none of these explain the frequently greater devastation of puerperal fever on the first obstetrical clinic, and that, on the contrary, some of these supposed causes are found to a greater degree in the second obstetric clinic.

This, and the pathological-anatomical findings in childbed fever, which bears the greatest resemblance to pyaemia in anatomists and surgeons, after wounding and impregnating their freshly injured bodies with rotten organic matter from corpses, led Dr. Semmelweis to the conviction that puerperal fever is likewise a pyemic process produced by the absorption of rotting organic matter from the inner lining of the uterus into the blood of the mother, and that the continued new introduction of such substances, especially on the first obstetric clinic, by the assistants and students must be accepted based on the daily dissection of corpses, but without excluding other modes of transfer of rotting organic constituents to the maternal organism, such as decomposed placental remnants, continual touching of sick and healthy pregnant and newly delivered women, and dissolution of fluids in other patients.

Following this idea, Dr. Semmelweis introduced careful hand-washing in a chlorine solution by any student or other investigators examining pregnant or recently delivered women, so as to eradicate any rotting organic atoms sticking to the fingers, even the smell of it, and, behold, the most brilliant success crowned this procedure for a full three years; namely, the mortality, which was 8.3% of recently delivered women on the first maternity clinic, is now the same as is observed in private practice and on the other maternity clinic, namely 2.3%.

Otherwise, the matter is further supported by the fact that, in the clinic for midwives there were often assistants who frequently examined corpses, and here, too, this disease claimed many victims that before the establishment of the general hospital (1784), until the establishment of an independent professorship for pathological anatomy, there was no so-called puerperal fever epidemic, and the mortality rate of the recently delivered women was not even 1%; but from the previously mentioned time until May, 1847, namely, until the commencement of chlorine washes, when the period of pathological anatomy was flowering, the total mortality rate on both clinics combined was 5.7%, but from then until last April of this year only 2.2% died. Further reasons for the endemic character of childbed fever are that the same does not prevail outside maternity clinics, that the seasons have no influence, and that it is the same after traumatic injury when no other epidemic disease is occurring, and also occurs in animals, but only sporadically, as it can be artificially created in the latter.

Puerperal fever, according to its above-mentioned nature, is, therefore, no more a contagious than a specific disease, but develops through the fact that an animal-organic substance, which has decayed, no matter which sick person, whether from a living organism or a cadaver, added to the blood of woman in childbirth, creates disintegration of the blood (pyemic), exudation, and third, the metastases. These substances are, however, added to the female organism by means of the examining finger, or by the use of equipment impregnated therewith, or also by the air which penetrates into the uterine cavity after birth, and which is impregnated with rotting substances, for which two striking examples are given. Therefore, prevention of this disease is possible by cleaning the fingers, the utensils and the air, whereupon only isolated cases of puerperal fever will result, like those from decaying decidua, or placenta remnants that have been left behind, through cracks and bruises on the cervix, and so on. As to the place where the absorption occurs, the lecturer identifies that accessible portion directly above the inner mouth of the uterus, which can be reached with the examining finger, which is covered by mucous membrane during pregnancy, loses its mucous membrane and is thus suitable for absorption and be capable of absorbing, but the vagina is covered by very thick epithelium and mucus. Most accessible is the uterine cavity during the first and second stage of labor, when examinations are most frequent; that explains why not only the mother, but also the child, perishes by the same great process of exudation at the onset of the disease, and why women who tarry for 2-3 days on the labor ward due to a delayed in the first and second stage of labor usually succumbed to virulent puerperal fever.

At the end of this lecture, Dr. Semmelweis announced that at one of the future general assemblies he wished to shed light on the objections that doctors Scanzoni and Seyfert raised in the Prague quarterly against his views on puerperal fever as expressed by Prof. Skoda in the Imperial Academy of Sciences, and, as a result, President Professor Rokitansky asked the society whether it was not generally inclined to enter into a discussion of this subject next time, given its importance, which was accepted.

REFERENCES CITED IN FOOTNOTES

József Antall (1968), "Welche Rolle spielten das Familienheim und dis Schule in der Entwicklung von Semmelweis Persönlichkeit?" *Communicationes de Historia Artis Medicinae*, 46-47: 95-126.

Isiah Berlin, "The Concept of Scientific History" in *Philosophical Analysis and History*, edited by William H, Dray, 5-53. New York, Harper & Row, 1966.

Alexander Bird (2010), "Eliminative Abduction: examples from medicine," *Studies in the History and Philosophy of Science* 41: 345-352.

Simon Blackburn (2017). *Truth* (London: Profile Books).

Herbert Butterfield (1965). *The Whig Interpretation of History* (New York: W. W. Norton Co.).

K. Codell Carter (1984), "Joseph's Skoda's relation to the Work of Ignaz Semmelweis," *Medizinhistorisches journal* 19: 335-47.

K. Codell Carter (1985), "Ignaz Semmelweis, Carl Mayrhofer, and the rise of germ theory," *Medical History*, 29: 33-53.

K. Codell Carter and George S. Tate (1991), "The earliest known account of Semmelweis's initiation of disinfection at Vienna's Allegemeines Krankenhaus," *Bulletin of the History of Medicine*, 65: 252-257.

K. Codell Carter (2003). *The rise of causal concepts of disease*. (London: Ashgate Publishing, Ltd.)

Robin G. Collingwood (1993). *The Idea of History*. (Oxford: Oxford University Press. Revised Edition. (Originally published in 1946)).

Robin G. Collingwood (1940). *An Essay on Metaphysics*. (Oxford: Clarendon Press. Reprinted by Martino Publishing, 2014).

Donald Davidson, *Causal Relations*, in *Causation*, Ernest Sosa and Michael Tooley (eds) (Oxford: Oxford University Press, 1993).

William Debbins (ed) (1965), *Essays in the Philosophy of History: R. G. Collingwood* (New York: McGraw-Hill Book Co.).

William Dray (1966). *Laws and Explanations in History* (Oxford: The Clarendon Press. First published 1957).

P. M. Dunn (2005), "Ignac Semmelweis (1818-1865) of Budapest and the prevention of puerperal fever," *Archives of Diseases in Childhood: Fetal and Neonatal Edition*, 50: 345-8.

Ganzinger K, Skopec M, Wyklicky, H (1981). *Festschrift für Erna Lesky zum 70. Geburtstag* (Vienna: Brüder Hollihnek).

Fielding Garrison (1929), *History of Medicine* (Philadelphia: W.B Saunders, 4th Ed.).

Donald Gillies (2005), "Hempelian and Kuhnian approaches in the philosophy of medicine: the Semmelweis case," *Studies in the History and Philosophy of Biological and Biomedical Sciences*, 36: 159-181.

Donald Gillies (2019), *Causality, Probability and Medicine* (Oxford: Routledge).

Nicholas Kadar (2019). "Rediscovering Ignaz Philipp Semmelweis 1818-1865," *American Journal of Obstetrics and Gynecology* 220: 26-39.

Nicholas Kadar (2020), "A note on Semmelweis's animal experiments and their historical significance," *Journal of the History of Medicine and Allied Sciences* (in press).

Nicholas Kadar and Russell D. Croft (2020), "Why Semmelweis's doctrine was rejected: evidence from the first publication of his results by Friedrich Wieger, and an Editorial commenting on the results," *British Journal of the History of Science* (available at doi:10.1017/S0007087420000229).

Paul Klemperer (1961a), "Notes on Carl von Rokitansky's Autobiography and Inaugural address," *Bulletin of the History of Medicine*, 35: 374-380.

Paul Klemperer (1961b), "Morbid Anatomy before and after Morgagni," *Bulletin of the New York Academy of Medicine*, 37:741-760.

Erna Lesky (1973), "Semmelweis IgnácraVonatkozó Iratok a Bécsi Egyetemi Levéltárbló," *Orvostörténeti Közlemények* (*Communicationes de Historia Artis Medicinae*) 66-68, 223-264

Irwine Loudon (2000). *The Tragedy of Childbed Fever* (Oxford: Oxford University Press).

Niklaus Mani (1966), Book Review: Erna Lesky: "Semmelweis und die Wiener Medizinische Schule," *Bulletin of the History of Medicine* 40:389-390.

Hans Meyerhoff (ed) (1959). Introduction in *The philosophy of history of our time* (New York: Doubeday Anchor Books).

Raymond Nickerson (1998), "Confirmation bias: A ubiquitous phenomenon in many guises," *Review of General Psychology* 2:175-220.

Sherwin B. Nuland (1979), "The Enigma of Semmelweis—an Interpretation, *Journal of the History of Medicine and Allied Sciences*," 34: 255-273.

Sherwin B. Nuland (2003). *The Doctors' Plague: Germs, Childbed Fever, and the Strange Story of Ignác Semmelweis* (New York: WW Norton & Company).

Michael Oakeshott (1962), "The activity of being an historian," in *Rationalism in Politics and Other Essays* (Indianapolis: LibertyPress).

Michael Oakeshott (1999). *On History and Other Essays* (Indianapolis: Liberty Fund, Inc, 1999, Originally published: Oxford: B. Blackwell, 1983)

Theodore G. Obenchain (2016). *Genius Belabored: Childbed Fever and the Tragic Life of Ignaz Semmelweis* (Tuscaloosa: The University of Alabama Press).

Karl Popper, "Has history any meaning," in *The Philosophy of History in our Time* edited by Hans Meyerhofff , 300-311. Doubleday Anchor Books, 1959.

Roy Porter (2002), *Blood and Guts: A Short History of Medicine* (New York: W.W. Norton & Company).

József Purgstaller (1843). *Bölcsészet Elemei* [Rudiments of Philosophy], available on line: http://real-eod.mtak.hu/3987/1/ABO_Z170885603_000840445.pdf

Alex Sakula (1981), "Joseph Skoda 1805-81: a centenary tribute to a pioneer of thoracic medicine," *Thorax* 36, 404-411.

David H. Sanford (2003). *If P, then Q: Conditionals and the foundation of reasoning* (London: Routledge, 2d ed.).

Rafael Scholl (2013), "Causal Inference, mechanisms, and the Semmelweis case," *Studies in the History and Philosophy of Science* 44: 66-76.

William J. Sinclair (1909), *Semmelweis: his life and his doctrine* (Manchester: Manchester University Press).

Frank G. Slaughter (1950), *Immortal Magyar* (New York: Henry Schuman).

Ernest Sosa and Michael Tooley (eds) (1993), *Causation* (Oxford: Oxford University Press).

A.J.P. Taylor (1948), *The Habsburg Monarchy:1809-1918* (Chicago: The University of Chicago Press).

Vladimir Vonka, "Causality in medicine: the case of tumours and viruses," *Philosophical Transactions of the Royal Society of London: Series B*, 335 (2000): 1831-1841

Fritz Schürer von Waldheim (1905), *Ignaz Philipp Semmelweis: Sein Leben und Wirken* (Wien u. Leipzig: Hartleben's Verlag).

W.H.Walsh, "Can History be objective?" in *The Philosophy of History in our Time* edited by Hans Meyerhofff , 216-224. New York: Doubleday Anchor Books, 1959.

Owen H. Wangensteen (1970), "Nineteenth century wound management of the parturient uterus and compound fracture: The Semmelweis-Lister priority controversy," *Bulletin. of the New York. Academy of Medicine*, 46, 565-596.

Timothy D. Wilson (2002), "Chapter 5: Knowing Why," in *Strangers to Ourselves: The Adaptive Unconscious* (Boston: Harvard University Press), 93-115.

David Wootton (2006). *Doctors Doing Harm Since Hippocrates* (Oxford: Oxford University Press).

INDEX

www.ingramcontent.com/pod-product-compliance
Lightning Source LLC
LaVergne TN
LVHW010718210926
848485LV00008B/1448/J
9781680539486